Digestive Diseases

Clinical Reviews

Formerly 'Survey of Digestive Diseases'
Founded in 1983 by T.S.N. Chen and R.K. Zetterman
Former Editor: S.R. Achem (1993–2000)

Official Journal of

EAGEN European Association for Gastroenterology and Endoscopy

KARGER 125 YEARS

Printed in Germany on acid-free and non-aging paper (ISO 9706) by Stückle Druck, Ettenheim

General Information

Digestive Diseases

ISSN Print Edition: 0257–2753
ISSN Online Edition: 1421–9875

Journal Homepage: www.karger.com/ddi

Publication Data: *Digestive Diseases* is published 6 times a year. Volume 33 with 6 issues appears in 2015.

Subscription Rates: Subscriptions run for a full calendar year. Prices are given per year.

Personal subscription:

Print or Online	Print+Online combined
CHF 320.00	CHF 368.00
EUR 267.00	EUR 306.00
USD 327.00	USD 375.00

postage and handling (added to print and print+online)
CHF 45.60 Europe, CHF 67.20 Overseas
EUR 38.40
USD 62.40

Institutional subscription:

Print or Online	Print+Online combined
CHF 2753.00	CHF 3166.00
EUR 2294.00	EUR 2683.00
USD 2809.00	USD 3230.00

postage and handling (added to print and print+online)
CHF 57.00 Europe, CHF 84.00 Overseas
EUR 48.00
USD 78.00

Discount subscription prices:
Please enquire about reduced rates for residents.

Back Volumes and Single Issues: Information on availability and prices of single print issues and print or electronic back volumes can be obtained from Customer Service at *service@karger.com.*

Bibliographic Indices: This journal is regularly listed in bibliographic services, including *Current Contents*® and PubMed/MEDLINE.

Subscription Orders:
Orders can be placed at agencies, bookstores, directly with the Publisher

S. Karger AG
Medical and Scientific Publishers
Allschwilerstrasse 10
CH–4009 Basel
Switzerland

t: +41 61 306 11 11
f: +41 61 306 12 34
e: karger@karger.com
w: www.karger.com

(for courier services only:
Allschwilerstrasse 10
CH–4055 Basel)

or further Karger offices
or representatives:

Germany
S. Karger GmbH
Postfach
79095 Freiburg
Deutschland
(Hausadresse: Wilhelmstrasse 20A,
79098 Freiburg)
t: +49 761 45 20 70
f: +49 761 45 20 714
e: information@karger.de
w: www.karger.de

Japan
Karger Japan, Inc.
Shiba Daimon Asahi Bldg. 2F
1-2-23 Shiba Daimon
Minato-ku
Tokyo 105-0012
Japan
t: +81 3 6435 6242
f: +81 3 6435 6244
e: publisher@karger.jp
w: www.karger.jp

USA
S. Karger Publishers, Inc.
26 West Avon Road
P.O. Box 529
Unionville, CT 06085
USA
Toll free: +1 800 828 5479
t: +1 860 675 7834
f: +1 860 675 7302
e: karger@snet.net

France
Enter & Read
Albertine Luginbuhl
23, rue du Départ, boite 37
75014 Paris
France
t: +33 (0) 6 81 04 76 85
e: albertineluginbuhl@orange.fr

South East Asia, China and Taiwan
Karger Regional Office (Malaysia)
Level 28-03-03A, PJ Exchange
No. 16A, Persiaran Barat
46050 Petaling Jaya
Selangor Darul Ehsan
Malaysia
t: +60 3 7962 0158
f: +60 3 7962 0001
e: service@karger.cn; r.chew@karger.cn

Karger China
51F Raffles City Centre
268 Xi Zang Middle Road
Huang Pu District
Shanghai 200001
P.R. China
t: +86 21 2312 7673
f: +86 21 2312 7777
e: service@karger.cn
r.chew@karger.cn
w: www.karger.cn

India, Bangladesh, Sri Lanka
Karger India
Plot No. 17, Yusuf Sarai Market
B.L. Glass Building, 2nd Floor
Sri Aurobindo Marg
New Delhi 110 016
India
t: +91 11 46029 633
f: +91 11 46029 634
c: +91 98 91052 128
e: r.kumar@kargerindia.com
w: www.karger.com

Change of Address:
Both old and new address should be sent to the subscription source.

KARGER

E-Mail karger@karger.com
www.karger.com

The Journal Home Page is available at:
www.karger.com/ddi

Digestive Diseases

Chronic Liver Diseases and Liver Cancer: An Update in 2015

12th Japan-Korea Liver Symposium

Osaka, Japan, July 5, 2015

Editors
Masatoshi Kudo, Osaka
Okio Hino, Tokyo
Soo-Ryang Kim, Kobe
Hyo-Suk Lee, Seoul
Kwang Hyub Han, Seoul
Young-Hwa Chung, Seoul

28 figures, 20 in color, and 19 tables, 2015

KARGER Basel · Freiburg · Paris · London · New York · Chennai · New Delhi · Bangkok · Beijing · Shanghai · Tokyo · Kuala Lumpur · Singapore · Sydney

S. Karger
Medical and Scientific Publishers
Basel · Freiburg · Paris · London ·
New York · Chennai · New Delhi ·
Bangkok · Beijing · Shanghai · Tokyo ·
Kuala Lumpur · Singapore · Sydney

Disclaimer
The statements, opinions and data contained in this publication are solely those of the individual authors and contributors and not of the publisher and the editor(s). The appearance of advertisements in the journal is not a warranty, endorsement, or approval of the products or services advertised or of their effectiveness, quality or safety. The publisher and the editor(s) disclaim responsibility for any injury to persons or property resulting from any ideas, methods, instructions or products referred to in the content or advertisements.

Drug Dosage
The authors and the publisher have exerted every effort to ensure that drug selection and dosage set forth in this text are in accord with current recommendations and practice at the time of publication. However, in view of ongoing research, changes in government regulations, and the constant flow of information relating to drug therapy and drug reactions, the reader is urged to check the package insert for each drug for any change in indications and dosage and for added warnings and precautions. This is particularly important when the recommended agent is a new and/or infrequently employed drug.

Printed on acid-free and non-aging paper (ISO 9706)
ISBN 978-3-318-05640-2
e-ISBN 978-3-318-05641-9

KARGER

E-Mail karger@karger.com
www.karger.com/ddi

Vol. 33, No. 6, 2015

Digestive Diseases

Contents

KARGER

E-Mail karger@karger.com
www.karger.com/ddi

Review Articles

Preface

Digestive Diseases

Dig Dis 2015;33:705–707
DOI: 10.1159/000439074

Chronic Liver Diseases and Liver Cancer: An Update in 2015

Masatoshi Kudo

Department of Gastroenterology and Hepatology, Kinki University School of Medicine, Osaka-Sayama, Osaka, Japan

The 12th Japan–Korea Liver Symposium was held in Osaka on July 5, 2015, in conjunction with the 6th Asia-Pacific Primary Liver Cancer Expert Meeting.

Nishida et al. [1] evaluated the antiviral response of triple therapy using peg-interferon, ribavirin and simeprevir (PEG-IFN/RBV/SMV) in the context of early reduction of viral load during treatment. They concluded that early viral response is a predictive factor for the achievement of sustained viral response 12, even in antiviral therapy with PEG-IFN/RBV/SMV. An extended treatment period should be used for patients who show detectable serum HCV-RNA at week 4.

Hasegawa et al. [2] evaluated cytokeratin-18M65 (CK-18M65) for distinguishing between simple steatosis and non-alcoholic steatohepatitis (NASH) against healthy individuals in the Japanese population. They concluded that serum CK-18M65 distinguished NASH from simple steatosis, but could not assess the severity of steatosis in non-alcoholic fatty liver disease patients on the grade of fibrosis in NASH patients with non-alcoholic steatohepatitis.

Sugimoto et al. [3] compared the characteristics of hypovascular and hypervascular well-differentiated hepatocellular carcinoma (HCC) in terms of tumor size, tumor markers [4–8] and detectability by imaging modalities [9–13]. They found that no difference was observed in tumor size and tumor markers between the 2 types of HCCs; however, the sensitivity of dynamic CT, contrast-enhanced ultrasonography with sonazoid and CT during arterial portography was significantly better in detecting hypervascular HCCs. However, detectability of hypovascular HCCs was inferior to the above-mentioned modalities, whereas hypovascular HCC could be diagnosed well by the hepatobiliary phase of MRI using gadolinium (Gd) ethoxybenzyl diethylenetriamine pentaacetic acid as a contrast agent [14].

Arizumi et al. [15] examined the efficacy and adverse events in 241 patients treated with sorafenib over a 6-year period at a single institution. They concluded that continuation of treatment with sorafenib for ≥90 days without deterioration of liver function was critical for obtaining the survival benefit of the patients if tumor response was determined as stable disease or higher.

Piscaglia et al. [16] evaluated the potential of MRI in the diagnosis of intrahepatic cholangiocellular carcinoma using ‘hepatocyte-specific’ Gd-based contrast agents. They concluded that MRI with hepatocyte-specific Gd-based contrast agents showed a pattern of malignancy in almost all intrahepatic cholangiocellular carcinoma, concurrently avoiding misdiagnosis with HCC.

Nishida et al. [17] studied epigenetic alterations that were responsible for HCC development [18] and identified the risk factors that were associated with DNA methylation in background liver tissue of non-B, non-C (NBNC) HCC patients. They concluded that background methylation was mostly associated with age in NBNC-HCC patients; some age-related methylation events could contribute to the emergence of NBNC-HCC in elderly individuals [19].

KARGER 125

E-Mail karger@karger.com
www.karger.com/ddi

0257–2753/15/0336–0705$39.50/0

Masatoshi Kudo, MD, PhD
Department of Gastroenterology and Hepatology
Kinki University School of Medicine
377-2 Ohno-Higashi, Osaka-Sayama, Osaka 589-8511 (Japan)
E-Mail m-kudo@med.kindai.ac.jp

Kudo et al. [20] developed the subclassification of BCLC B intermediate stage HCCs by modifying the Blondi's subclassification. They state that the Kinki criteria subclassified BCLC B stage into 3 substages: B1 (Child-Pugh score 5–7, within up-to-7 criteria), B2 (Child-Pugh score 5–7, beyond up-to-7 criteria) and B3 (Child-Pugh score 8, 9 and any tumor status). They emphasized that the stratification ability of this criteria is more efficient and easier to apply to clinical practice than the original Blondi's subclassification. Furthermore, the concept of treatment indication ranges from curative intent (B1), palliative treatment (B2) and no treatment (B3) subgroups, which is relevant to clinical practice of BCLC B patients [21].

Minami et al. [22] described that cone-beam CT angiography is capable of providing more information than the standard 2D angiography in visualizing HCCs and targeting tumors through precise microcatheter placement in close proximity to HCCs. They concluded that cone-beam CT has the potential to significantly impact the practice of interventional radiology.

Kudo et al. [23] described the significance of establishing general rules, a nationwide follow-up survey and clinical practice guidelines for liver cancer in Japan. They emphasized that both the evidence-based and consensus-based treatment algorithms for HCC are used to complement each other in clinical practice in Japan [24].

Nishida et al. [25] reported the molecular mechanism and prediction of sorafenib chemoresistance in human HCC. To date, a number of studies have examined the underlying mechanisms involved in the response to sorafenib and trials have been performed to overcome the acquisition of drug resistance. They stated that the activation of an escape pathway from RAF/MEK/ERK possibly results in chemoresistance. In addition, there are several features of HCCs indicating sorafenib resistance, such as epithelial mesenchymal transition and positive stem cell markers.

Kudo et al. [26] overviewed the challenges of clinical practice and research on HCC regarding tumor markers, imaging, pathological diagnosis, treatment strategy, staging system and subclassification. They also described the difference in the practice pattern between Japan and Western countries.

Finally, I strongly believe that this special issue 'Chronic Liver Diseases and Liver Cancer: An Update in 2015' will be beneficial and invaluable for all readers who specialize in liver diseases and HCC.

References

1 Nishida N, Iwanishi M, Minami T, Chishina H, Arizumi T, Takita M, Kitai S, Yada N, Ida H, Hagiwara S, Minami Y, Ueshima K, Sakurai T, Kitano M, Kudo M: Early viral response predicts the efficacy of antiviral triple therapy with simeprevir, peg-interferon, and ribavirin in patients infected with hepatitis C virus genotype 1. Dig Dis 2015;33:708–714.

2 Hasegawa Y, Kim SR, Hatae T, Ohta M, Fujinami A, Sugimoto K, Kim KI, Imoto S, Tohyama M, Kim SK, Ikura Y, Kudo M: Usefulness of cytokeratin-18M65 in diagnosing non-alcoholic steatohepatitis in Japanese population. Dig Dis 2015;33:715–720.

3 Sugimoto K, Kim SR, Imoto S, Tohyama M, Kim SK, Matsuoka T, Kudo M, Yano Y, Hayashi Y: Characteristics of hypovascular vs. hypervascular well-differentiated hepatocellular carcinoma smaller than 2cm – focus on tumor size, markers and imaging detectability. Dig Dis 2015;33:721–727.

4 Kudo M: Biomarkers and personalized sorafenib therapy. Liver Cancer 2014;3:399–404.

5 Shao YY, Hsu CH, Cheng AL: Predictive biomarkers of antiangiogenic therapy for advanced hepatocellular carcinoma: where are we? Liver Cancer 2013;2:93–107.

6 Kudo M: Alpha-fetoprotein-L3: useful or useless for hepatocellular carcinoma? Liver Cancer 2013;2:151–152.

7 Song P, Gao J, Inagaki Y, Kokudo N, Hasegawa K, Sugawara Y, Tang W: Biomarkers: evaluation of screening for and early diagnosis of hepatocellular carcinoma in Japan and China. Liver Cancer 2013;2:31–39.

8 Toyoda H, Kumada T, Tada T, Sone Y, Kaneoka Y, Maeda A: Tumor markers for hepatocellular carcinoma: simple and significant predictors of outcome in patients with HCC. Liver Cancer 2015;4:126–136.

9 Murakami T, Tsurusaki M: Hypervascular benign and malignant liver tumors that require differentiation from hepatocellular carcinoma: key points of imaging diagnosis. Liver Cancer 2014;3:85–96.

10 Ichikawa T, Sano K, Morisaka H: Diagnosis of pathologically early HCC with EOB-MRI: experiences and current consensus. Liver Cancer 2014;3:97–107.

11 Kudo M, Matsui O, Izumi N, Iijima H, Kadoya M, Imai Y, Okusaka T, Miyayama S, Tsuchiya K, Ueshima K, Hiraoka A, Ikeda M, Ogasawara S, Yamashita T, Minami T, Yamakado K; Liver Cancer Study Group of Japan: JSH consensus-based clinical practice guidelines for the management of hepatocellular carcinoma: 2014 update by the liver cancer study group of Japan. Liver Cancer 2014; 3:458–468.

12 Minami Y, Kudo M: Imaging modalities for assessment of treatment response to nonsurgical hepatocellular carcinoma therapy: contrast-enhanced US, CT, and MRI. Liver Cancer 2015;4:106–114.

13 Ichikawa S, Ichikawa T, Motosugi U, Sano K, Morisaka H, Enomoto N: Was hypervascular hepatocellular carcinoma visible on previous gadoxetic acid-enhanced magnetic resonance images? Liver Cancer 2015;4:154–162.

14 Kudo M: Early hepatocellular carcinoma: definition and diagnosis. Liver Cancer 2013;2: 69–72.

15 Arizumi T, Ueshima K, Iwanishi M, Chishina H, Kono M, Takita M, Kitai S, Inoue T, Yada N, Hagiwara S, Ida H, Minami Y, Sakurai T, Nishida N, Kitano M, Kudo M: Real-life clinical practice with sorafenib in advanced hepatocellular carcinoma: a single-center experience second analysis. Dig Dis 2015;33:728–734.

16 Piscaglia F, Iavarone M, Galassi M, Vavassori S, Renzulli M, Forzenigo LV, Granito A, Salvatore V, Sangiovanni A, Golfieri R, Colombo M, Bolondi L: Cholangiocarcinoma in cirrhosis: value of hepatocyte specific magnetic resonance imaging. Dig Dis 2015;33:735–744.

17 Nishida N, Iwanishi M, Minami T, Chishina H, Arizumi T, Takita M, Kitai S, Yada N, Ida H, Hagiwara S, Minami Y, Ueshima K, Sakurai T, Kitano M, Kudo M: Hepatic DNA methylation is affected by hepatocellular carcinoma risk in patients with and without hepatitis virus. Dig Dis 2015;33:745–750.
18 Nishida N, Kudo M: Alteration of epigenetic profile in human hepatocellular carcinoma and its clinical implications. Liver Cancer 2014;3:417–427.
19 Effendi K, Yamazaki K, Fukuma M, Sakamoto M: Overexpression of leucine-rich repeat-containing G protein-coupled receptor 5 (LGR5) represents a typical Wnt/β-catenin pathway-activated hepatocellular carcinoma. Liver Cancer 2014;3:451–457.
20 Kudo M, Arizumi T, Ueshima K, Sakurai T, Kitano M, Nishida N: Subclassification of BCLC B (intermediate)-stage hepatocellular carcinoma and treatment strategies: modified Bolondi's subclassification (Kinki Criteria). Dig Dis 2015;33:751–758.
21 Kudo M: Recent advances in bioinformatics reveal the molecular heterogeneity of hepatocellular carcinoma. Liver Cancer 2014;3:68–70.
22 Minami Y, Murakami T, Kitano M, Sakurai T, Nishida N, Kudo M: Cone-Beam CT angiography for hepatocellular carcinoma: current status. Dig Dis 2015;33:759–764.
23 Kudo M, Kitano M, Sakurai T, Nishida N: General rules for the clinical and pathological study of primary liver cancer, nationwide follow-up survey, and clinical practice guidelines: the outstanding achievements of the liver cancer study group of Japan. Dig Dis 2015;33:765–770.
24 Raoul JL, Park JW, Kang YK, Finn RS, Kim JS, Yeo W, Polite BN, Chao Y, Walters I, Baudelet C, Lencioni R: Using modified RECIST and alpha-fetoprotein levels to assess treatment benefit in hepatocellular carcinoma. Liver Cancer 2014;3:439–450.
25 Nishida N, Kitano M, Sakurai T, Kudo M: Molecular mechanism and prediction of sorafenib chemoresistance in human hepatocellular carcinoma. Dig Dis 2015;33:771–779.
26 Kudo M, Kitano M, Sakurai T, Nishida N: Challenges of clinical research on hepatocellular carcinoma. Dig Dis 2015;33:780–790.

Original Article

Digestive Diseases

Dig Dis 2015;33:708–714
DOI: 10.1159/000439075

Early Viral Response Predicts the Efficacy of Antiviral Triple Therapy with Simeprevir, Peg-Interferon and Ribavirin in Patients Infected with Hepatitis C Virus Genotype 1

Naoshi Nishida Mina Iwanishi Tomohiro Minami Hirokazu Chishina Tadaaki Arizumi Masahiro Takita Satoshi Kitai Norihisa Yada Hiroshi Ida Satoru Hagiwara Yasunori Minami Kazuomi Ueshima Toshiharu Sakurai Masayuki Kitano Masatoshi Kudo

Department of Gastroenterology and Hepatology, Kinki University School of Medicine, Osaka-Sayama, Osaka, Japan

Key Words

Chronic hepatitis C · Simeprevir · NS3/4 protease inhibitors · Interferon · Response-guided therapy

Abstract

Objectives: Triple therapy using peg-interferon, ribavirin and simeprevir (PEG-IFN/RBV/SMV) has reportedly resulted in high-sustained virological response (SVR) rates in patients with chronic hepatitis C (CHC), especially in naïve cases and relapsers to prior PEG-IFN/RBV therapy. Here, we retrospectively analyzed the antiviral response associated with a triple regimen, in the context of early reduction of viral load during treatment. ***Methods:*** Forty-six CHC patients with HCV genotype 1b were treated with PEG-IFN/RBV/SMV triple therapy: 20 were naïve cases, 12 were relapsers and 14 were non-responders to prior PEG-IFN/RBV therapy. We evaluated rapid virological response (RVR), complete early virological response (EVR), viral clearance at the end of the treatment (EOT) and at 12 weeks after the EOT (SVR12). In addition, we quantified the serum HCV-RNA on the 1st day and the 7th day after initiating treatment. ***Results:*** Multivariate analysis revealed that response to prior treatment was identified as an independent factor for achieving SVR12 after triple therapy ($p = 0.0005$). The achievement of serum HCV-RNA <2 $\log_{10}$ IU/ml on day 7, RVR, EVR and EOT were associated with SVR12 ($p = 0.0050$, $p = 0.0002$, $p = 0.0009$ and $p = 0.0002$, respectively). ***Conclusions:*** Rapid decline of HCV is a predictive factor for the achievement of SVR12, even in antiviral triple therapy with PEG-IFN/RBV/SMV. An extended treatment period should be applied for patients who show detectable serum HCV-RNA at week 4.

Introduction

Chronic hepatitis C (CHC) is one of the leading causes of liver cirrhosis worldwide and a major etiology for the emergence of hepatocellular carcinoma (HCC) [1]. Recent advancements in antiviral therapy for CHC allow us to have more treatment options, including triple therapy using peg-interferon (PEG-IFN), ribavirin (RBV) and NS3 protease inhibitors [2, 3]. Although IFN-free regimens are becoming more common, IFN-based regimens are still widely used for antiviral therapy of hepatitis C virus (HCV) because they can have a suppressive effect on the emergence of HCC and are associated with lower

Naoshi Nishida, MD
Department of Gastroenterology and Hepatology
Kinki University School of Medicine
337-2 Ohno-Higashi, Osaka-Sayama, Osaka 589-8511 (Japan)
E-Mail naoshi@med.kindai.ac.jp

risk for developing virus mutations that are resistant to direct-acting antivirals (DAAs) [4, 5].

Simeprevir (SMV) is a second-generation non-structural protein (NS) 3/4 protease inhibitor with a better safety profile than first-generation NS3/4 protease inhibitors; the latter, for example, are known to induce severe drug-induced eruptions [6]. Several reports have suggested that antiviral triple therapy with PEG-IFN, RBV and SMV (PEG-IFN/RNV/SMV) have shown powerful antiviral effects on HCV [2, 3, 7–9]. For example, 88.6% of patients in a study demonstrated sustained virological response 12 weeks after treatment end (SVR12) in treatment-naïve cases with HCV genotype 1 infection and high viral load (HCV-RNA ≥5 $\log_{10}$ IU/ml) [10]. In addition, SVR12 was achieved in 95.9% of the patients who relapsed prior to receiving PEG-RFN and RBV combination therapy (PEG-IFN/RBV) and in 52.8% of prior nonresponders (NRs) [11]. It has also been reported that PEG-IFN/RBV/SMV triple therapy may be effective after 24 weeks, compared to that after the standard 48-week regimen used in conventional PEG-IFN/RBV treatment [7]. Due to the potential efficacy of a PEG-IFN-based triple regimen, a treatment plan using triple therapy with SMV for 12 weeks, followed by additional administration of PEG-IFN/RBV for 12 weeks (SMV12/PR12), has been recommended for the treatment of naïve patients and prior relapsers. For prior NRs, an additional 36 weeks of administration of PEG-IFN/RBV after the initial 12 weeks of administration of 3 agents was also admitted (SMV12/PR36) [12].

Based on these findings, we conducted a retrospective analysis of the antiviral response of patients treated with a triple regimen of PEG-IFN/RBV/SMV, especially in the context of early reduction of viral load after treatment was initiated. For this purpose, we examined viral load intensively in the early phase of treatment.

Materials and Methods

Patients

Forty-six CHC patients infected with HCV genotype 1b were treated with PEG-IFN/RBV/SMV triple therapy between December 2013 and March 2015. All patients had a viral load of ≥5 $\log_{10}$ IU/ml before the treatment. The median age of the patients was 64.5 years, with a range of 33–81 years. Eighteen were men and 28 were women. Twenty-five patients were treated with PEG-IFN α-2a (Pegasys®, Chugai Pharmaceutical Co., Ltd., Tokyo, Japan), and 21 patients were administered PEG-IFN α-2b (PegIntron®, Merck Sharp & Dohme, Whitehouse Station, N.J., USA). Twenty-one showed *IL-28B* T/T genotype (rs8099917) and 12 were T/G, and data were missing for 13 patients. HCV with a mutation at the core amino acid 70 (core 70) was detected in 9 patients, while a wild mutation for core 70 was noted in 9 patients (data were missing for 19 patients). Of 46 patients, 20 were naïve cases, 12 were relapsers and 14 were NRs to prior treatment with PEG-IFN/RBV.

Assessment of Viral Response

Serum HCV-RNA was quantified at week 4 and week 12 to evaluate rapid virological response (RVR) and complete early virological response (EVR), respectively. Similarly, we analyzed viral clearance at the end of the treatment (EOT) and 12 weeks after the EOT (SVR12). In order to evaluate the decline of serum HCV-RNA during the initial treatment phase, we also quantified the serum HCV-RNA on the 1st day and the 7th day after treatment was initiated. Quantification was performed using the COBAS® TaqMan® HCV Auto Assay System (Roche, USA; lower limit of quantification, 1.2 $\log_{10}$ IU/ml).

Statistical Analysis

The Pearson's chi-square test or the Fisher's exact test was used to compare categorical variables. For comparisons of continuous variables, the Wilcoxon rank-sum test and the Student t test were applied. All p values were 2-sided, and p value of <0.05 was considered statistically significant. All statistical analyses were performed using JMP version 9.0 software (SAS Institute Inc., Cary, N.C., USA).

Results

Alteration of Serum HCV-RNA during Treatment and Response to Prior Antiviral Therapy

Among the 46 patients treated with PEG-IFN/RBV/SMV, 20 were naïve cases, 12 were relapsers and 14 were NRs to prior dual therapy with PEG-IFN/RBV. Naïve cases and prior relapsers received treatment for 24 weeks (SMV12/PR12). Among 14 prior NRs, 2 patients who showed EVR (undetectable HCV-RNA at week 12) during PEG-IFN/RBV/SMV therapy received treatment with SMV12/PR36, while 7 NRs with EVR received SMV12/PR12 treatment. Five patients did not achieve serum HCV-RNA level <1.2 $\log_{10}$ IU/ml between the 12th week and the 24th week, and therapy was therefore discontinued before the completion of 24th week. Figure 1 illustrates the changes in serum HCV-RNA levels during and after treatment. We evaluated undetectable serum HCV-RNA 12 weeks after the completion of treatment (SVR12) in 42 patients, and of these, 30 achieved SVR12. Among 20 naïve cases, 1 patient showed EOT but did not achieve SVR12 (relapse) after the completion of triple therapy, and 1 patient showed breakthrough (BT) in the 20th week, although the HCV-RNA level was below the lower limit of quantification. Among 12 patients who showed relapse after the prior treatment, one relapsed again after triple therapy with PEG-IFN/RBV/SMV. Conversely, re-

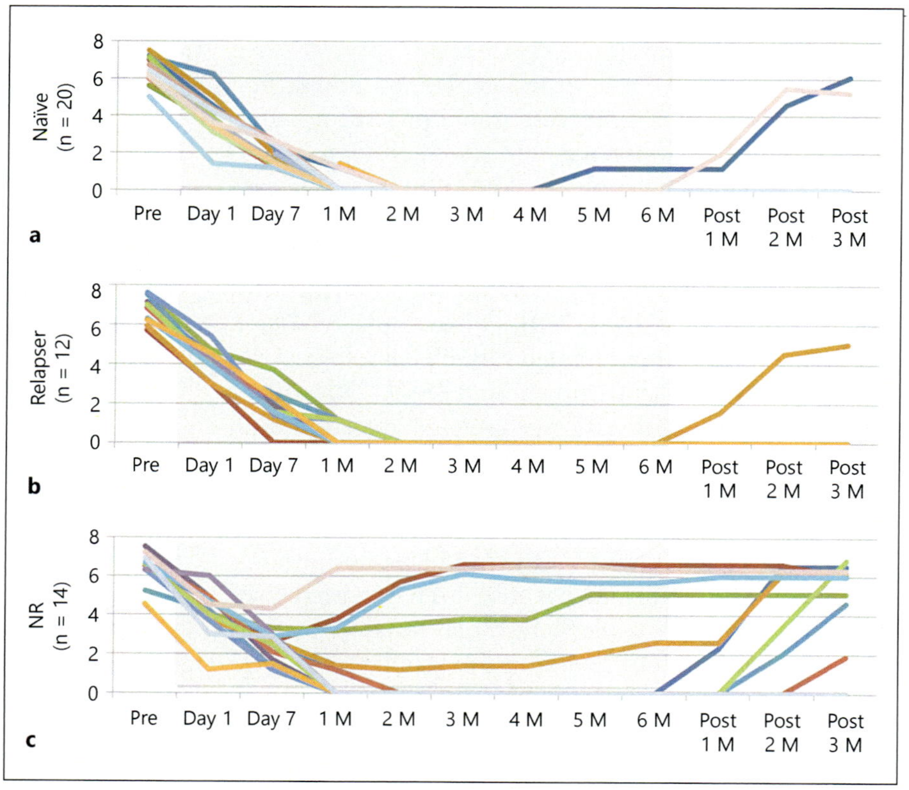

Fig. 1. The alteration of serum HCV-RNA level during and after the treatment with PEG-IFN/RBV/SMV. The alteration of serum HCV-RNA level in naïve cases (**a**), in relapsers to prior PEG-IFN/RBV treatment (**b**) and prior NRs (**c**). The vertical showed HCV-RNA level ($\log_{10}$ IU/ml). The gray rectangle showed the periods under antiviral therapy. Two of 14 prior NRs received antiviral therapy for 48 weeks. M = Month.

lapse after triple therapy was observed in 4 of 14 NRs for prior treatment, and serum HCV-RNA did not reach the undetectable level (NR) in 5 patients.

Figure 2 shows the proportion of patients who achieved a defined virological response at each stage of the PEG-IFN/RBV/SMV treatment. Virological responses after initiation of treatment were defined as follows: achievement of HCV-RNA decline ≥2 $\log_{10}$ IU/ml from baseline (2 log drop on day 1), HCV-RNA level <2 $\log_{10}$ IU/ml on day 7 (<2 log on day 7), undetectable serum HCV-RNA at week 4 (RVR), undetectable serum HCV-RNA at week 12 (EVR) and undetectable serum HCV-RNA at the EOT. Although not statistically significant, prior NRs had a lower achievement rate than naïve cases and prior relapsers for 2 log drop on day 1, <2 log on day 7 and RVR, suggesting that the decline of serum HCV-RNA was slower in prior NRs than in naïve cases and prior relapsers. In addition, EVR, EOT and SVR12 rates were significantly lower in prior NRs than in naïve cases and prior relapsers. All naïve cases, all relapsers and 63% of NRs achieved EVR ($p = 0.0020$). In all, 94% of naïve cases, all relapsers and 64% of NRs achieved EOT ($p = 0.0151$). Finally, 88% of naïve cases, 92% of relapsers and 35% of NRs achieved SVR12 ($p = 0.0014$).

Pretreatment Conditions and Response to PEG-IFN/RBV/SMV Treatment

We analyzed the association between background conditions and response after PEG-IFN/RBV/SMV treatment. Among the background factors, *IL-28B* genotype was associated with viral response to PEG-IFN/RBV/SMV treatment in all phases of treatment, and T/T genotype was associated with good antiviral response (fig. 3a). Of special importance, significant associations were observed for EVR and SVR12, where 95% of T/T and 64% of T/G cases achieved EVR ($p = 0.0367$; fig. 3a), and 85% of T/T and 45% of T/G cases showed SVR12 ($p = 0.0377$; fig. 3a and table 1). On the other hand, no associations were observed between the presence of core 70 mutations and antiviral response (fig. 3b).

Among the 42 patients who were evaluated for SVR12, 31 were analyzed for *IL-28B* genotype. Twenty were of genotype T/T and 11 were of T/G genotype. Among the 20 patients with T/T genotype, 17 achieved SVR12 (85%), 2 showed BT/relapse (10%) and 1 was considered as NR (5%) for triple therapy. On the other hand, among the 11 patients carrying T/G genotype, 5 (45%), 2 (18%) and 4 patients (36%) showed SVR12, BT/relapse and NR, respectively ($p = 0.0437$; fig. 3c).

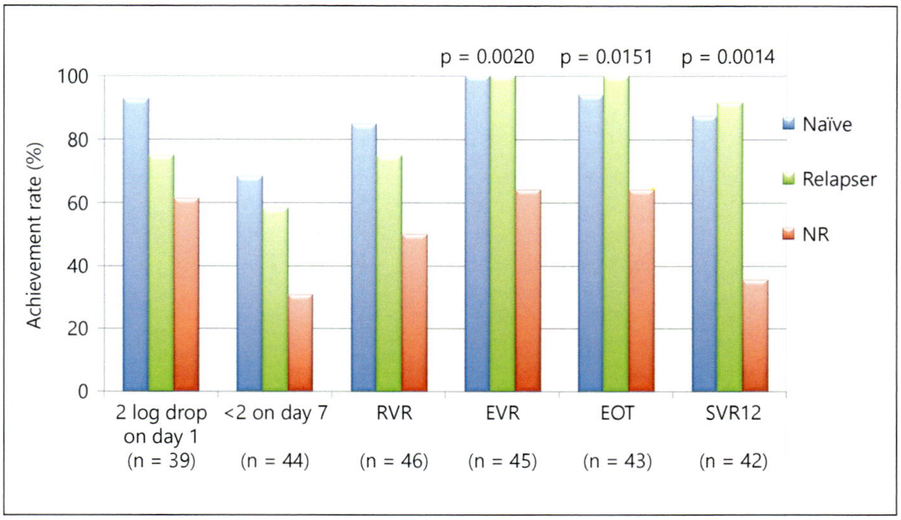

Fig. 2. Percentage of the patients who achieved a defined virological response at each stage of the PEG-IFN/RBV/SMV treatment: 2 log drop on day 1, decrease of serum HCV-RNA is 2 log_{10} IU/ml or grater from base line on day 1 of the treatment; <2 on day 7, serum HCV-RNA level <2 log_{10} IU/ml; RVR, undetectable serum HCV-RNA at week 4; EVR, undetectable serum HCV-RNA at week 12; EOT, undetectable serum HCV-RNA at the EOT; SVR12, undetectable serum HCV-RNA 12 weeks after the EOT. p values are calculated by the Pearson's chi-square test.

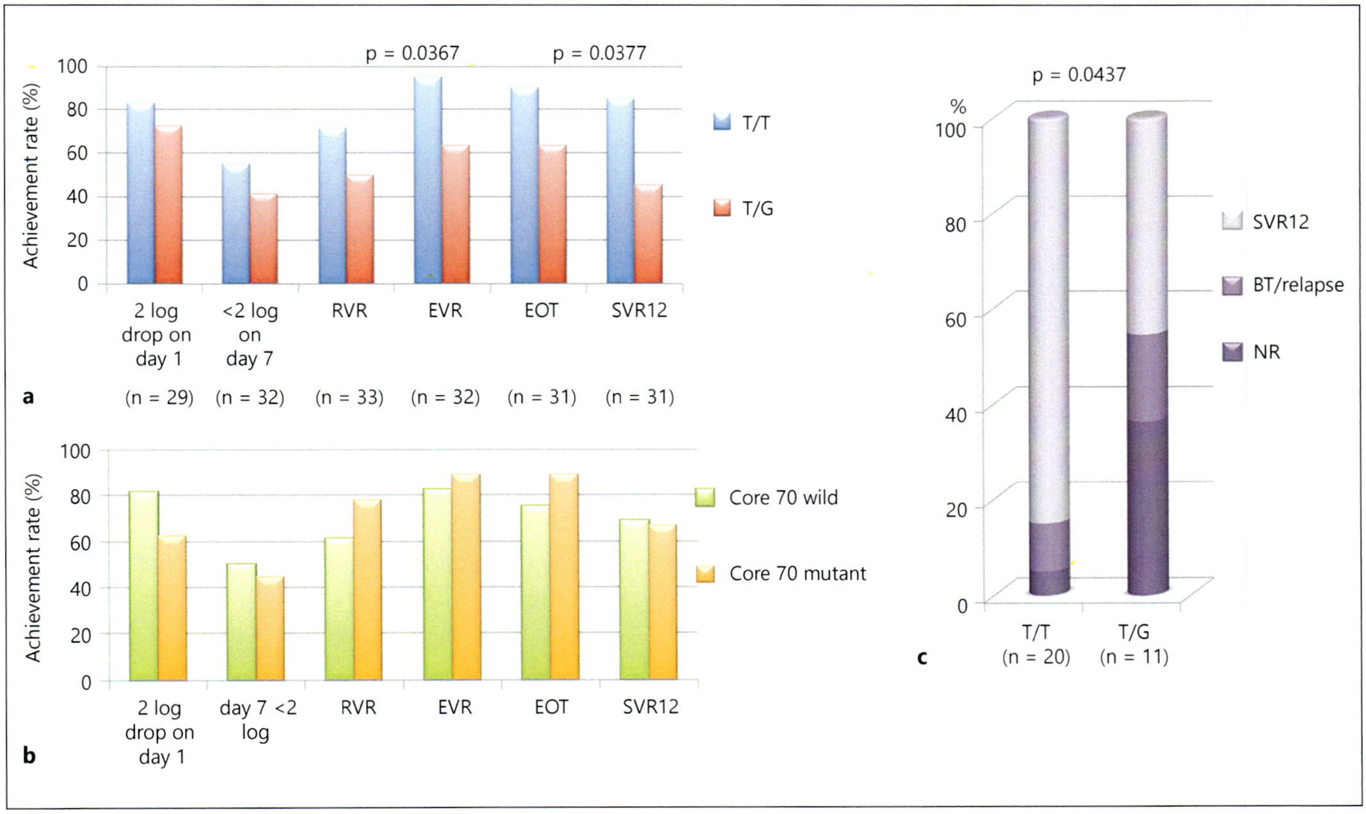

Fig. 3. The association between *IL-28B* genotype, presence of HCV with core 70 mutation and antiviral response of the PEG-IFN/RBV/SMV. Achievement rate in each phase of treatment is shown in the context of *IL-28B* genotype (**a**) and presence or absence of HCV core 70 mutation (**b**). p values are calculated by the Fisher's exact test. Association between *IL-28B* genotype and responses to PEG-IFN/RBV/SMV treatment at 12 weeks after the EOT are shown (**c**). Among 20 patients with T/T genotype, 17 achieved SVR12, 2 showed BT/relapse and 1 was a NR. On the other hand, among the 11 patients carrying T/G genotype, 5, 2 and 4 patients showed SVR12, BT/relapse and NR, respectively. p values are calculated by the Pearson's chi-square test.

Dig Dis 2015;33:708–714
DOI: 10.1159/000439075

Table 1. Pretreatment conditions that are associated with achievement of SVR at 12 weeks post treatment

	Univariate			Multivariate	
	SVR12 (+) (n = 30)	SVR12 (–) (n = 12)	p value	OR (95% CI)	p value
Age, years					
Mean (95% CI)	64 (60–68)	57 (51–63)	0.0655		
Sex					
Male/female	12/18	5/7	1.0000		
IL-28B[1]					
TT/TG	17/5	3/6	**0.0377**	2.72 (0.25–30.0)	0.3951
Core 70[2]					
Wild/mutant	11/6	5/3	1.0000		
Prior treatment[3]					
Naïve or relapse/NR	25/5	3/9	**0.0006**	37.4 (4.30–875.7)	**0.0005**

[1] Genotype is determined at rs8099917.
[2] Presence (mutant) or absence (wild) of HCV with the mutant core 70 mutation.
[3] Response to prior treatment with PEG-INF and RBV. Naïve, a patient without prior treatment. Relapser, a patient who showed undetectable HCV-RNA at the end of the treatment but detectable HCV-RNA during follow-up. NR, a patient who never showed undetectable HCV-RNA. p values <0.05 are shown in bold.

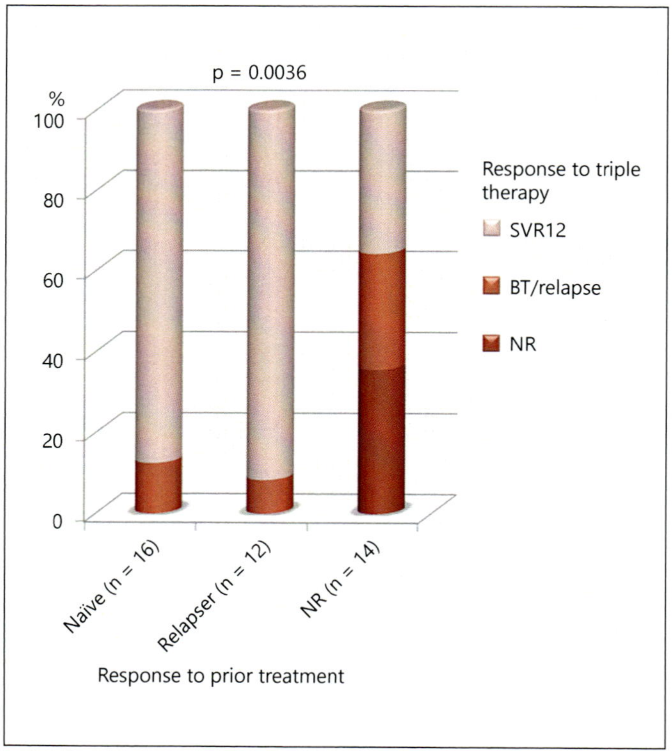

Fig. 4. The association between response to prior treatment with PEG-IFN/RBV and achievement of SVR12 after triple therapy. Among 16 naïve cases, 14 showed SVR12. Similarly, 11 of 12 prior relapsers achieved SVR12. On the other hand, only 5 showed SVR12 among 15 prior NRs. p values are calculated by the Pearson's chi-square test.

Figure 4 represents the association between response to prior treatment with PEG-IFN/RBV and achievement of SVR12 after triple therapy. Among 16 naïve cases, 14 had SVR12 (88%). Similarly, 11 of 12 prior relapsers achieved SVR12 (92%). On the other hand, only 5 showed SVR12 (36%) among 15 prior NRs (p = 0.0036; fig. 4). We also conducted multivariate analysis using *IL-28B* genotype and response to prior treatment as co-variables. Response to prior treatment was identified as an independent factor for achieving SVR12 after triple therapy (naïve or relapser vs. NR, p = 0.0005, OR 37.4, 95% CI 4.30–875.7; table 1).

EVR and Achievement of SVR12 in PEG-IFN/RBV/SMV Treatment

We also analyzed the association between an early antiviral response for PEG-IFN/RBV/SMV triple therapy and achievement of SVR12 (fig. 5). Reduction of 2 log on day 1, <2 log on day 7, RVR, EVR and EOT were associated with SVR12 (this was statistically significant for <2 log on day 7, RVR, EVR and EOT with p values 0.0050, 0.0002, 0.0009 and 0.0002, respectively). All patients who failed to achieve EVR and EOT resulted in relapse, BT or NR, after PEG-IFN/RBV/SMV triple therapy. Among 21 patients who showed <2 log on day 7, 19 achieved SVR12 (positive predictive value (PPV 91%)). Ten patients failed to achieve SVR12 among 19 patients that did not demonstrate <2 log on day 7 (negative predictive value (NPV 53%)). Similarly, among 29 patients who showed RVR, 16

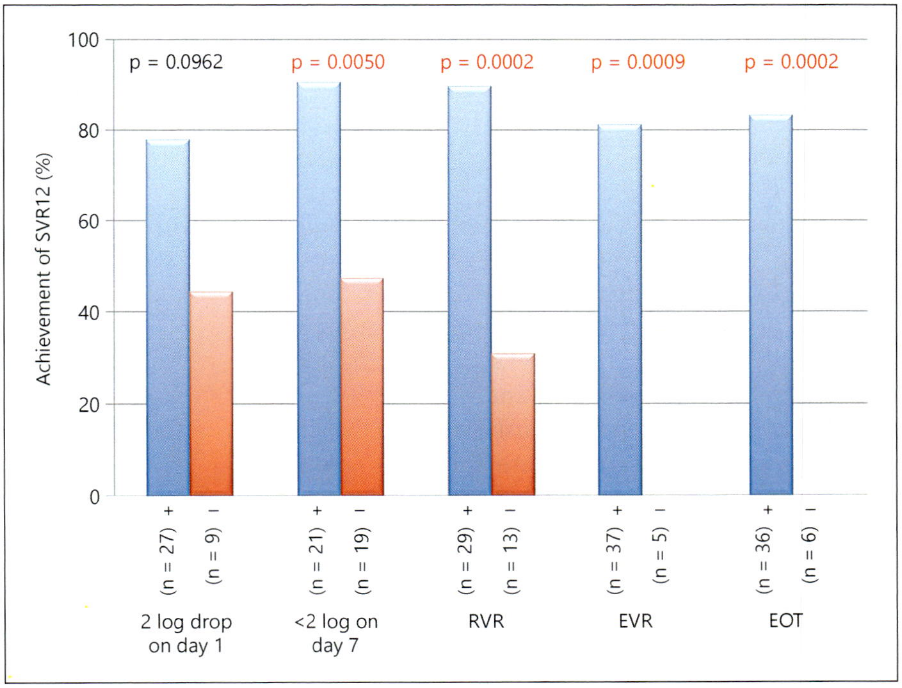

Fig. 5. The association between antiviral responses for PEG-IFN/RBV/SMV during treatment and achievement of subsequent SVR12. Achievements of 2 log drop on day 1, <2 log on day 7, RVR, EVR and EOT are significantly associated with that of SVR12. p values are calculated by the Fisher's exact test.

achieved SVR12 (PPV 90%), and 9 failed to achieve SVR12 among 13 patients without RVR (NPV 69%). The 16 naïve cases and the 12 prior relapsers could be evaluated for SVR12. Of these, 3 patients failed to achieve SVR12. Notably, in 2 of 3 naïve/prior relapsers who did not show SVR12 after triple therapy, HCV-RNA was detectable at week 4, although it was below the lower limit of quantification. On the other hand, among 5 patients who were NRs to prior treatment and achieved SVR12 after triple therapy, all showed undetectable HCV-RNA at week 4, although 2 of 5 patients received SMV12/PR36.

Discussion

Recently, IFN-free regimens for CHC using DAAs have been shown to achieve high SVR rates, even for patients who did not respond to IFN-based therapy [13]. On the other hand, there are still concerns about IFN-free regimens, and emergence of mutated HCV resistant to DAAs could affect the efficacy of future antiviral treatments [14, 15]. Furthermore, in contrast to IFN-based therapy, the suppressive effect of DAAs on HCC development is still unclear [5]. Therefore, for treatment of CHC with genotype 1b and high viral load, triple therapy using a second-generation protease inhibitor, PEG-IFN, and RBV should still be considered for naïve cases, as well as for re-treatment cases without a history of protease inhibitor use. This approach is supported by the most recent guidelines for the management of HCV infection proposed by the Japan Society of Hepatology (http://www.jsh.or.jp/medical/guidelines/jsh_guidlines/hepatitis_c). However, failure of a triple regimen could also lead to the emergence of resistant viruses for NS3/4A protease inhibitors, which is mainly attributable to the amino acid substitution at D168 [14, 16]. From this point of view, predicting relapse in the early phase of treatment is important so the length of treatment can be extended such as SMV12/PR36 regimen. In this study, we demonstrated that EVR is a predictive factor for the achievement of SVR12, even in antiviral therapy with PEG-IFN/RBV/SMV.

In concordance with earlier studies, our data also show that a genotype of *IL-28B* and responses to prior treatment are significantly associated with the achievement of SVR12 following triple regimen therapy [8]. Response to prior treatment is identified as a particularly important independent factor for SVR12. It is also well documented that response to prior IFN-based treatment reflects the antiviral effect of IFN that is critical for achieving SVR, even for patients treated with PEG-IFN/RBV/SMV [9, 11]. Our data also show that SVR12 rates are high in naïve cases and prior relapsers, reaching 88 and 92%, respectively.

On the other hand, 2 naïve cases and 1 relapser failed to achieve SVR12. Two of the 3 patients who were naïve

DOI: 10.1159/000439075

or prior relapsers, and failed to achieve SVR12, revealed detectable HCV-RNA at week 4, although the level was below the lower limit of quantification. On the other hand, 5 prior NRs achieved SVR12 following triple therapy; all of them showed RVR. Therefore, we further analyzed the viral response of each phase of treatment in the context of achieving SVR12. We found that, in addition to EVR and EOT, the degree of HCV decline on day 7 and the rate of undetectable HCV at week 4 were both significantly associated with subsequent achievement of SVR12 (PPV and NPV for SVR12 were 91 and 53% for achievement of <2 log on day 7, and 90 and 69% for RVR, respectively). It has been previously reported that the decline of serum HCV-RNA at treatment week 4 was a good marker of SVR in patients with HCV genotype 1/high viral load, who received treatment with response-guided PEG-IFN plus RBV combination therapy [17]. This evidence suggests that EVR is a surrogate marker of the antiviral effect of IFN, and this could affect antiviral response even in treatment with PRG-IFN/RBV/SMV.

In this report, we showed that rapid decline of HCV and undetectable HCV-RNA at week 4 of treatment, should be a surrogate marker for predicting SVR12 in triple therapy using REG-IFN/RBV/SMV in both naïve/prior relapser and in NRs. From this point of view, extension of the treatment period should be considered for patients with detectable serum HCV-RNA at week 4, even in naïve cases and prior relapsers to PEG-IFN/RBV.

Acknowledgments

This work was supported in part by Grant-in-Aid for Scientific Research (KAKENHI: 24590997) from the Japanese Society for the Promotion of Science (N. Nishida) and a grant from the Smoking Research Foundation (N. Nishida).

Disclosure Statement

The authors have no conflicts of interest to disclose.

References

1 Kim do Y, Han KH: Epidemiology and surveillance of hepatocellular carcinoma. Liver Cancer 2012;1:2–14.

2 Fried MW, Buti M, Dore GJ, Flisiak R, Ferenci P, Jacobson I, Marcellin P, Manns M, Nikitin I, Poordad F, Sherman M, Zeuzem S, Scott J, Gilles L, Lenz O, Peeters M, Sekar V, De Smedt G, Beumont-Mauviel M: Once-daily simeprevir (TMC435) with pegylated interferon and ribavirin in treatment-naïve genotype 1 hepatitis C: the randomized PILLAR study. Hepatology 2013;58:1918–1929.

3 Forns X, Lawitz E, Zeuzem S, Gane E, Bronowicki JP, Andreone P, Horban A, Brown A, Peeters M, Lenz O, Ouwerkerk-Mahadevan S, Scott J, De La Rosa G, Kalmeijer R, Sinha R, Beumont-Mauviel M: Simeprevir with peginterferon and ribavirin leads to high rates of SVR in patients with HCV genotype 1 who relapsed after previous therapy: a phase 3 trial. Gastroenterology 2014;146:1669–1679.e3.

4 Pockros PJ: Advances in newly developing therapy for chronic hepatitis C virus infection. Front Med 2014;8:166–174.

5 Hiramatsu N, Oze T, Takehara T: Suppression of hepatocellular carcinoma development in hepatitis C patients given interferon-based antiviral therapy. Hepatol Res 2015;45:152–161.

6 Asselah T, Marcellin P: Second-wave IFN-based triple therapy for HCV genotype 1 infection: simeprevir, faldaprevir and sofosbuvir. Liver Int 2014;34(suppl 1):60–68.

7 Jacobson IM, Dore GJ, Foster GR, Fried MW, Radu M, Rafalsky VV, Moroz L, Craxi A, Peeters M, Lenz O, Ouwerkerk-Mahadevan S, De La Rosa G, Kalmeijer R, Scott J, Sinha R, Beumont-Mauviel M: Simeprevir with pegylated interferon alfa 2a plus ribavirin in treatment-naive patients with chronic hepatitis C virus genotype 1 infection (QUEST-1): a phase 3, randomised, double-blind, placebo-controlled trial. Lancet 2014;384:403–413.

8 Manns M, Marcellin P, Poordad F, de Araujo ES, Buti M, Horsmans Y, Janczewska E, Villamil F, Scott J, Peeters M, Lenz O, Ouwerkerk-Mahadevan S, De La Rosa G, Kalmeijer R, Sinha R, Beumont-Mauviel M: Simeprevir with pegylated interferon alfa 2a or 2b plus ribavirin in treatment-naive patients with chronic hepatitis C virus genotype 1 infection (QUEST-2): a randomised, double-blind, placebo-controlled phase 3 trial. Lancet 2014;384:414–426.

9 Kumada H, Hayashi N, Izumi N, Okanoue T, Tsubouchi H, Yatsuhashi H, Kato M, Rito K, Komada Y, Seto C, Goto S: Simeprevir (TMC435) once daily with peginterferon-α-2b and ribavirin in patients with genotype 1 hepatitis C virus infection: the CONCERTO-4 study. Hepatol Res 2015;45:501–513.

10 Hayashi N, Izumi N, Kumada H, Okanoue T, Tsubouchi H, Yatsuhashi H, Kato M, Ki R, Komada Y, Seto C, Goto S: Simeprevir with peginterferon/ribavirin for treatment-naïve hepatitis C genotype 1 patients in Japan: CONCERTO-1, a phase III trial. J Hepatol 2014;61:219–227.

11 Izumi N, Hayashi N, Kumada H, Okanoue T, Tsubouchi H, Yatsuhashi H, Kato M, Ki R, Komada Y, Seto C, Goto S: Once-daily simeprevir with peginterferon and ribavirin for treatment-experienced HCV genotype 1-infected patients in Japan: the CONCERTO-2 and CONCERTO-3 studies. J Gastroenterol 2014;49:941–953.

12 Takehara T: Simeprevir for the treatment of chronic hepatitis C genotype 1 infection. Expert Rev Anti Infect Ther 2014;12:909–917.

13 Schinazi R, Halfon P, Marcellin P, Asselah T: HCV direct-acting antiviral agents: the best interferon-free combinations. Liver Int 2014; 34(suppl 1):69–78.

14 Halfon P, Locarnini S: Hepatitis C virus resistance to protease inhibitors. J Hepatol 2011; 55:192–206.

15 Poveda E, Wyles DL, Mena A, Pedreira JD, Castro-Iglesias A, Cachay E: Update on hepatitis C virus resistance to direct-acting antiviral agents. Antiviral Res 2014;108:181–191.

16 Lenz O, Verbinnen T, Fevery B, Tambuyzer L, Vijgen L, Peeters M, Buelens A, Ceulemans H, Beumont M, Picchio G, De Meyer S: Virology analyses of HCV isolates from genotype 1-infected patients treated with simeprevir plus peginterferon/ribavirin in phase IIb/III studies. J Hepatol 2015;62:1008–1014.

17 Editors of the Drafting Committee for Hepatitis Management Guidelines: The Japan Society of Hepatology: guidelines for the management of hepatitis C virus infection: first edition, May 2012, the Japan Society of Hepatology. Hepatol Res 2013;43:1–34.

Original Article

Digestive Diseases

Dig Dis 2015;33:715–720
DOI: 10.1159/000439076

Usefulness of Cytokeratin-18M65 in Diagnosing Non-Alcoholic Steatohepatitis in Japanese Population

Yutaka Hasegawa[a] Soo Ryang Kim[b] Takashi Hatae[d] Mitsuhiro Ohta[e] Aya Fujinami[e] Kayo Sugimoto[c] Ke Ih Kim[c] Susumu Imoto[b] Madoka Tohyama[b] Soo Ki Kim[f] Yoshihiro Ikura[g] Masatoshi Kudo[h]

[a]Department of Pharmacy, Division of Medical Technology, Shinko Hospital, [b]Departments of Gastroenterology and [c]Pharmacy, Kobe Asahi Hospital, [d]Educational Center for Clinical Pharmacy and [e]Medical Biochemistry, Kobe Pharmaceutical University, Kobe, [f]Department of Gastroenterology and Hepatology, Kyoto University, Kyoto, [g]Department of Pathology, Takatsuki General Hospital, Takatsuki, Osaka, and [h]Department of Gastroenterology and Hepatology, Kinki University, School of Medicine, Osaka-Sayama, Osaka, Japan

Key Words

Non-alcoholic steatohepatitis · Non-alcoholic fatty liver disease · CK-18M65 · Serum biomarker · Japanese population

Abstract

Objective: The aim of this study was to evaluate cytokeratin-18M65 (CK-18M65) for distinguishing between simple steatosis (SS) and non-alcoholic steatohepatitis (NASH) against healthy individuals (HIs) in Japanese population. ***Methods:*** The serum from 24 HIs, 21 patients with SS and 20 patients with NASH were examined. Serum CK-18M65 was measured by enzyme-linked immunosorbent assay. ***Results:*** Aspartate aminotransferase was significantly different between NASH patients and HIs with $p < 0.0001$ (SS patients and HIs: $p < 0.0001$), as was alanine aminotransferase between NASH patients and HIs with $p < 0.0001$ (SS patients and HIs: $p < 0.0001$). Serum CK-18M65 increased in a stepwise fashion in HIs and also in SS and NASH patients. Multivariate logistic regression analysis revealed that NASH could be diagnosed with the use of CK-18M65 alone ($p = 0.0285$, OR 1.0038, 95% CI 1.0004–1.0073). At the optimal cut-off level of 548 U/l, CK-18M65 had an AUC value of 0.7369, 60.00% sensitivity and 85.70% specificity. In patients with NASH, no significant difference was observed between low fibrosis (Stage 0–1, 794.30 ± 454.41, n = 10) and high fibrosis (Stage 2–3, 809.70 ± 641.43, n = 10; $p = 0.5967$) and between slight steatosis (<33%, 512.89 ± 229.65, n = 9) and moderate steatosis (≥33%, 655.13 ± 480.78, n = 32) in patients with non-alcoholic fatty liver disease (NAFLD; $p = 0.7647$) with the use of CK-18M65. ***Conclusion:*** Serum CK-18M65 distinguished NASH from SS, but could not assess the severity of steatosis in NAFLD patients or the grade of fibrosis in NASH patients in Japanese population.

Introduction

Non-alcoholic fatty liver disease (NAFLD), one of the most common and chronic liver diseases worldwide [1], comprises simple steatosis (SS) and non-alcoholic steatohepatitis (NASH); the latter is considered the hepatic manifestation of metabolic syndrome.

KARGER 125

E-Mail karger@karger.com
www.karger.com/ddi

0257–2753/15/0336–0715$39.50/0

Soo Ryang Kim, MD
Department of Gastroenterology
Kobe Asahi Hospital
3-5-25 Bououji-cho, Nagata-ku, Kobe, 653-0801 (Japan)
E-Mail asahi-hp@arion.ocn.ne.jp

Table 1. Participant characteristics and univariate analysis in distinguishing between SS and NASH against HIs

	NASH	SS	HI	p value		
				NASH vs. SS	NASH vs. HI	SS vs. HI
Age, years	58.80±14.59	47.52±14.38	57.46±6.88	0.0843	0.8896	0.0217
Sex, male/female	8/12	15/6	4/20			
CK-18M65	802.00±541.08	454.29±215.46	211.38±92.19	0.0255	<0.0001	<0.0001
AST	65.85±58.17	41.86±31.63	18.83±3.63	0.0620	<0.0001	<0.0001
ALT	80.30±59.24	70.48±76.53	16.08±3.87	0.5737	<0.0001	<0.0001
γ-GTP	64.00±59.66	95.67±108.18	25.96±15.50	0.9966	0.0001	0.0012
TC	214.70±31.39	183.38±48.02	220.50±34.84	0.0896	0.8256	0.0256
TG	176.40±74.54	161.67±104.72	121.92±58.94	0.6153	0.0440	0.3234
HDL-C	58.75±39.97	50.90±15.49	66.04±18.76	0.9338	0.0256	0.0090
GLU	117.25±46.26	97.00±20.22	90.42±9.55	0.2323	0.0209	0.4825
Hb	14.28±1.88	14.85±1.46	13.30±1.03	0.5244	0.0806	0.0019
PLT	20.86±4.88	23.19±5.40	25.17±4.79	0.5656	0.0344	0.3293

Among individuals with NAFLD, SS is a benign condition, but NASH can progress to fibrosis, cirrhosis and ultimately hepatocellular carcinoma [2–6]. The precise mechanism of NASH is poorly understood [7], although its etiology is attributed to insulin resistance and oxidative stress. Although used in the detection of NAFLD, imaging techniques such as CT and ultrasonography are not adequate for distinguishing between SS and NASH [7, 8]. Steatosis, ballooning, inflammation and fibrosis are major histopathological features of NASH [7, 9]. Liver biopsy used in the diagnosis of SS and NASH is an invasive procedure that requires hospitalization [10, 11] and may sometimes cause major complications like hemorrhage [10].

Therefore, there is an urgent need to develop simple, non-invasive serum biomarkers that can accurately distinguish between NASH and SS in patients and in healthy individuals (HIs), and to identify the grade of liver fibrosis in patients with NASH and the severity of steatosis in patients with NAFLD [7, 10].

Several serum biomarkers such as cytokeratin-18 (CK-18M65 and CK-18M30) and CD14 have been used to distinguish between SS and NASH [12–14]. CK-18M65 as a serum biomarker measuring overall cell death including cleaved and uncleaved caspase can distinguish NASH from SS patients, versus HIs in European populations, and has been useful in differentiating the severity of hepatic steatosis in patients with NAFLD and the degree of fibrosis in patients with NASH [7].

The aim of this study is to assess the clinical value of CK-18M65 as a tool for distinguishing between SS and NASH, and assessing the grade of fibrosis in patients with NASH and the severity of steatosis in patients with NAFLD in Japanese population.

Patients and Methods

NAFLD was diagnosed by abdominal ultrasonography and CT. The serum from 41 patients who underwent liver biopsy at Kobe Asahi Hospital were analyzed: 20 patients (8 men, 12 women, 58.80 ± 14.59 years) with NASH, 21 patients (15 men, 6 women 47.52 ± 14.38 years) with SS and 24 HIs (4 men, 20 women, 57.46 ± 6.88 years) who did not undergo biopsy (table 1).

Patients with evidence of excessive alcohol use (≥80 g/week) and other causes of liver disease (hepatitis B, hepatitis C, autoimmune liver disease and drug- or toxin-induced liver steatosis) were excluded from the study.

The study protocol was approved by the Clinical Research Ethics Committee of Kobe Asahi Hospital.

Liver Histology

Liver biopsy specimens were fixed in formalin and embedded in paraffin, sectioned and stained with hematoxylin-eosin for routine histological analysis and evaluation by 2 expert hepatopathologists (S.R.K. and Y.I.). Fibrosis in NASH was evaluated using the Azan-Mallory stain.

Histological grading and staging of NAFLD were scored according to the system reported by Kleiner et al. [9]. Steatosis was classified by degree: F0 <5%, 5%≤ F1 <33%, 33%≤ F2 <66% and F3 ≥66%. Fibrosis was staged from 0 to 4: 0 = no fibrosis, 1 = perisinusoidal or periportal fibrosis, 2 = perisinusoidal and portal/periportal fibrosis, 3 = bridging fibrosis and 4 = cirrhosis.

Clinical and Laboratory Assessments

Serum samples were examined for aspartate aminotransferase (AST; in IU/l), alanine aminotransferase (ALT; in IU/l), gamma-glutamyl transpeptidase (γ-GTP; in IU/l), total cholesterol (TC; in mg/dl), triglyceride (TG; in mg/dl), high-density lipoprotein cholesterol (HDL-C; in mg/dl), glucose (GLU; in mg/dl), hemoglobin (Hb; in g/dl) and platelets (PLT; in 10^4/μl).

The serum level of CK-18M65 was measured using the M65 ELISA kit (PEVIVA, Stockholm, Sweden) according to the manufacturers' instructions [15] to determine the stages of fibrosis from low (F0–F1, n = 10) to high (F2–F3, n = 10) in patients with NASH and the severity of steatosis from slight to moderate in patients with NAFLD.

Statistical Analysis

Variables are shown as means ± SD or percentages. Serum biomarkers in HIs as well as in patients with SS and NASH were compared using the Kruskal–Wallis and the Steel–Dwass tests.

Receiver operating characteristics (ROCs) was calculated for the cut-off value of NASH. The cut-off value was analyzed by the ROC curve. A p value of <0.05 was considered significant. Variables with a p value of <0.1 in the univariate analysis were included in stepwise multivariate logistic regression analysis. Variables with a p value of <0.05 in multivariate analysis were considered statistically significant. A multivariate logistic regression analysis was conducted to adjust for variables associated with NASH. Statistical analyses were computed with the use of Ekuseru-Toukei 2012 (Social Survey Research Information Co., Ltd., Japan).

Results

Participant Characteristics and Univariate Analysis in Distinguishing between SS and NASH Patients against HIs

The clinical and laboratory characteristics of the participants are described in table 1. Serum CK-18M65, AST, ALT, TG and GLU were high in SS and NASH patients compared with HIs. On the other hand, serum PLT was low in SS and NASH patients than in HIs. Significant differences were observed in the values of AST: NASH vs. HI (p < 0.0001) and SS vs. HI (p < 0.0001); ALT: NASH vs. HI (p < 0.0001) and SS vs. HI (p < 0.0001); γ-GTP: NASH vs. HI (p = 0.0001) and SS vs. HI (p = 0.0012); TC: SS vs. HI (p = 0.0256); TG: NASH vs. HI (p = 0.0440); HDL-C: NASH vs. HI (p = 0.0256) and SS vs. HI (p = 0.0090); GLU: NASH vs. HI (p = 0.0209); Hb: SS vs. HI (p = 0.0019); PLT: NASH vs. HI (p = 0.0344). Also, CK-18M65 was significantly different among patients with NASH and SS and HIs (NASH vs. SS: p = 0.0255; NASH vs. HI: p < 0.0001; SS vs. HI: p < 0.0001).

Diagnosis of NASH Using Serum Biomarkers in NAFLD Patients

Multivariate logistic regression analysis revealed that NASH could be diagnosed by CK-18M65 alone (p = 0.0285, OR 1.0038, 95% CI 1.0004–1.0073; table 2).

To determine the predictive discriminating value of the serum biomarkers for the detection of NASH, ROC analysis was performed.

At the optimal cut-off level of 548 U/l, CK-18M65 demonstrated an AUC value of 0.7369, 60.00% sensitivity and 85.70% specificity in detecting NASH (fig. 1).

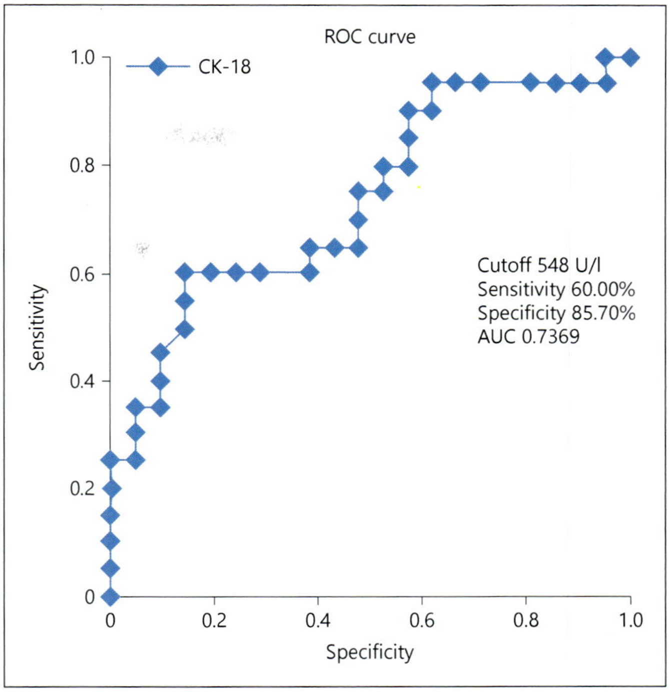

Fig. 1. Prediction of NASH by ROC analysis.

Table 2. Multivariate logistic regression analysis associated with NASH

	OR	95% CI	p value
Age	1.0827	1.0126–1.1577	0.0200
CK-18M65	1.0038	1.0004–1.0073	0.0285
AST	1.0099	0.9928–1.0272	0.2585
TC	1.0224	0.9960–1.0495	0.0975

At a cut-off value of 548 U/l for CK-18M65, PPV and NPV in the diagnosis of NASH and SS demonstrated 80.00 and 69.23%, respectively, with a significant difference between them (p = 0.0036; fig. 1; data not shown).

Relation of CK-18 in NASH Fibrosis Grade and in NAFLD Steatosis Grade

Fibrosis in 20 NASH patients ranged from stages 0 to 4: stage 0 (n = 0), stage 1 (n = 10), stage 3 (n = 6) and stage 4 (n = 4). No significant difference was found in the stages of fibrosis between low 0–1 (794.30 ± 454.41, n = 10) and high 2–3 (809.70 ± 641.43, n = 10; p = 0.5967; fig. 2). Also, no significant difference was observed between mild steatosis in 2 patients (<33%, 419.50 ± 12.02) and moderate steatosis in 18 patients (≥33%, 884.50 ± 555.04).

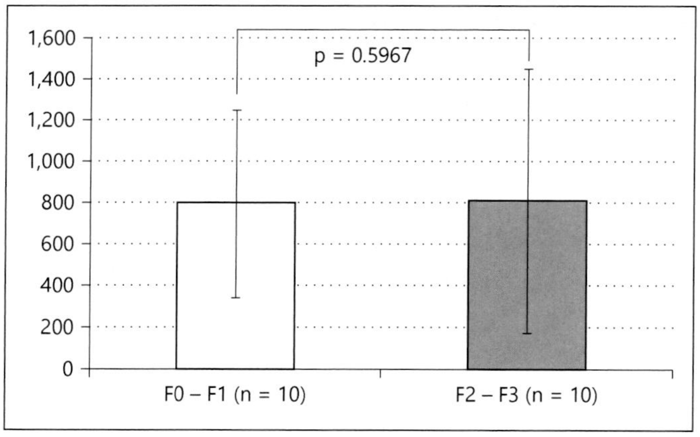

Fig. 2. Relation of CK-18–NASH fibrosis grade.

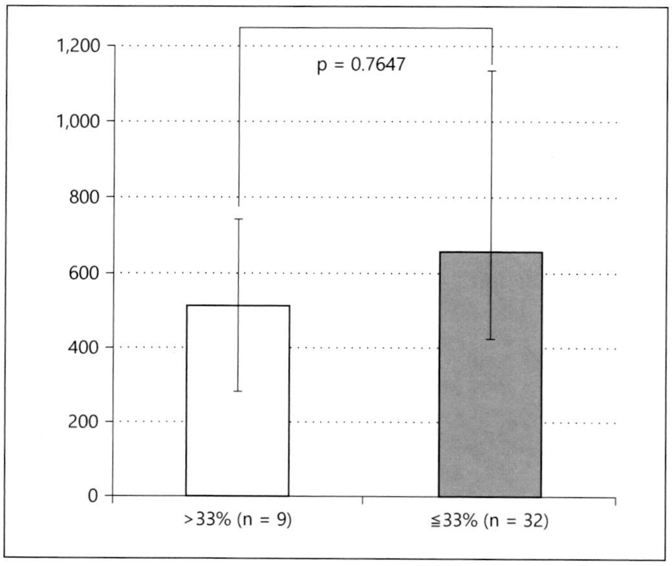

Fig. 3. Relation of CK-18–NAFLD steatosis grade.

Because of the small number of patients with NASH, the severity of steatosis analyzed in NAFLD patients (n = 41) was mild (<33% in 9 patients, 512.89 ± 222.65) and moderate (>33% in 32 patients, 655.13 ± 480.78), with no significant difference between them (fig. 3).

Discussion

NAFLD comprises a spectrum of chronic diseases ranging from SS to NASH [16, 17].

Distinguishing between SS and NASH is crucial because the latter increases the risk of the progression of the disease to cirrhosis and hepatocellular carcinoma [18].

In distinguishing intermediate from minimal fibrosis – a prerequisite to clinical decision-making – fibrosis serum biomarkers such as collagen IV and hyaluronic acid do so only slightly, but are not useful in distinguishing NASH from SS [7].

At present, liver biopsy is the only reliable procedure for distinguishing SS from NASH and assessing the severity of liver damage and grading fibrosis [19]. It is, however, an invasive procedure that requires hospitalization.

There is, therefore, an urgent need to develop simple, non-invasive serum biomarkers that can accurately distinguish between NASH and SS vs. HIs and to identify the grade of liver fibrosis in patients with NASH and the severity of steatosis in patients with NAFLD [7, 10].

In this study, the level of serum AST was significantly higher in NASH patients than in HIs, and that of serum ALT was significantly different among HIs as well as SS and NASH patients; however, no significant difference was observed between SS and NASH. TG, AST and ALT levels increase significantly with the progression of NAFLD [20]; AST levels are significantly higher in NASH than in non-NASH patients [12]; the PLT count decreases in patients with NASH or severe fibrosis [21–23]. On the other hand, no statistical difference in platelet count has been found between non-NASH and NASH patients [24]. Nonetheless, these laboratory data are not adequate enough for differentiating NASH from SS; our results were compatible with those of Feldstein et al. [12] but not with those of Kashyap et al. [20].

Hepatocyte apoptosis has been recognized as a mechanism of liver injury that may also contribute to fibrogenesis [7]. Apoptosis is an active ATP-dependent process that contributes to the maintenance of tissue homeostasis under normal physiological conditions [25]. CK-18 is an intracellular protein mainly produced by necrosis and apoptosis of cells of epithelial origin including hepatocytes, and is a useful serum biomarker that reflects cell death [26]. Recently, serum CK-18M65 released in NAFLD patients in the process of the cellular death has been proposed as a possible serum biomarker of NASH [27, 28]. The increased serum levels of CK-18 fragments, in some clinical cohorts of obese patients or those with insulin resistance, are associated with hepatocyte injury, inflammation and fibrosis [29].

Of the 2 kinds of CK-18 (CK-18M65 and CK-18M30), CK-18M65 has been mentioned as a serum biomarker of overall cell death, including cleaved and uncleaved caspase, that can distinguish between NASH and SS patients and HIs in a European population [7] and can assess the severity of steatosis in patients with NAFLD and the grade of fibrosis in patients with NASH [7]. Nonetheless, the clinical utility of CK-18 has been tested in 139 NAFLD patients in a European population [12], whereas there are various differences between the Japanese and the Europeans: body weight, diet, life style and genes related to disease occurrence.

Therefore, we aimed at evaluating CK-18M65 as a laboratory index for distinguishing among HIs and patients with SS and NASH and at assessing the severity of steatosis and the grade of fibrosis in patients with NASH in a Japanese population. The results demonstrated that serum CK-18M65 increased in a stepwise fashion in HIs and in patients with SS and NASH and that the value of CK-18M65 was significant ($p = 0.0036$) in distinguishing between SS and NASH.

By multivariate logistic regression analysis, CK-18M65 was independently associated with NASH ($p = 0.0058$, OR 1.00481, 95% CI 1.0014–1.0081). The ROC curve and the area under ROC curve were used to assess the utility of parameters in the diagnosis of NASH [29]. Moreover, in comparing between NASH and SS, the level of CK-18M65 detected by M65 ELISA, around 548 U/l, correctly predicted NASH with a sensitivity of 60.00%, a specificity of 85.7% and an AUC value of 0.7369 (fig. 1). These results suggest the efficacy of CK-18M65 as a serum biomarker in distinguishing patients with NASH from those with SS versus the HIs and its use as a non-invasive serum biomarker of NASH, replacing the burden of liver biopsies. It could not, however, assess the severity of steatosis and the stages of fibrosis.

The limits of this study lie in the paucity of the number of patients and the ethnic differences between the European and the Japanese populations.

Because of the limitations of our single-center study and the relatively small number of non-NASH patients, further studies in a large-scale, multicenter and validation cohort are needed to confirm our conclusions.

Acknowledgment

We are indebted to Ms Mika Matsui for assistance in the preparation of the manuscript.

Disclosure Statement

The authors have no financial conflicts of interest.

References

1 Farrell GC, Larter CZ: Nonalcoholic fatty liver disease: from steatosis to cirrhosis. Hepatology 2006;43(2 suppl 1):S99–S112.

2 Ekstedt M, Franzén LE, Mathiesen UL, Thorelius L, Holmqvist M, Bodemar G, et al: Long-term follow-up of patients with NAFLD and elevated liver enzymes. Hepatology 2006; 44:865–873.

3 Wong VW, Wong GL, Choi PC, Chan AW, Li MK, Chan HY, et al: Disease progression of non-alcoholic fatty liver disease: a prospective study with paired liver biopsies at 3 years. Gut 2010;59:969–974.

4 Younossi ZM, Jarrar M, Nugent C, Randhawa M, Afendy M, Stepanova M, et al: A novel diagnostic biomarker panel for obesity-related nonalcoholic steatohepatitis (NASH). Obes Surg 2008;18:1430–1437.

5 Wong VW, Chan HL, Hui AY, Chan KF, Liew CT, Chan FK, et al: Clinical and histological features of non-alcoholic fatty liver disease in Hong Kong Chinese. Aliment Pharmacol Ther 2004;20:45–49.

6 Wong VW, Hui AY, Tsang SW, Chan JL, Tse AM, Chan KF, et al: Metabolic and adipokine profile of Chinese patients with nonalcoholic fatty liver disease. Clin Gastroenterol Hepatol 2006;4:1154–1161.

7 Joka D, Wahl K, Moeller S, Schlue J, Vaske B, Bahr MJ, et al: Prospective biopsy-controlled evaluation of cell death biomarkers for prediction of liver fibrosis and nonalcoholic steatohepatitis. Hepatology 2012;55: 455–464.

8 Saadeh S, Younossi ZM, Remer EM, Gramlich T, Ong JP, Hurley M, et al: The utility of radiological imaging in nonalcoholic fatty liver disease. Gastroenterology 2002;123:745–750.

9 Kleiner DE, Brunt EM, Van Natta M, Behling C, Contos MJ, Cummings OW, et al: Design and validation of a histological scoring system for nonalcoholic fatty liver disease. Hepatology 2005;41:1313–1321.

10 Shen J, Chan HL, Wong GL, Choi PC, Chan AW, Chan HY, et al: Non-invasive diagnosis of non-alcoholic steatohepatitis by combined serum biomarkers. J Hepatol 2012;56:1363–1370.

11 Cadranel JF, Rufat P, Degos F: Practices of liver biopsy in France: results of a prospective nationwide survey. For the Group of Epidemiology of the French Association for the Study of the Liver (AFEF). Hepatology 2000; 32:477–481.

12 Feldstein AE, Wieckowska A, Lopez AR, Liu YC, Zein NN, McCullough AJ: Cytokeratin-18 fragment levels as noninvasive biomarkers for nonalcoholic steatohepatitis: a multicenter validation study. Hepatology 2009;50:1072–1078.

13 Diab DL, Yerian L, Schauer P, Kashyap SR, Lopez R, Hazen SL, et al: Cytokeratin 18 fragment levels as a noninvasive biomarker for nonalcoholic steatohepatitis in bariatric surgery patients. Clin Gastroenterol Hepatol 2008;6:1249–1254.

14 Imajo K, Yoneda M, Ogawa Y, Wada K, Nakajima A: Microbiota and nonalcoholic steatohepatitis. Semin Immunopathol 2014;36: 115–132.

15 Bantel H, Lügering A, Heidemann J, Volkmann X, Poremba C, Strassburg CP, et al: Detection of apoptotic caspase activation in sera from patients with chronic HCV infection is associated with fibrotic liver injury. Hepatology 2004;40:1078–1087.

16 Torres DM, Williams CD, Harrison SA: Features, diagnosis, and treatment of nonalcoholic fatty liver disease. Clin Gastroenterol Hepatol 2012;10:837–858.

17 Cusi K: Role of obesity and lipotoxicity in the development of nonalcoholic steatohepatitis: pathophysiology and clinical implications. Gastroenterology 2012;142:711–725.

18 Chalasani N, Younossi Z, Lavine JE, Diehl AM, Brunt EM, Cusi K, et al: The diagnosis and management of non-alcoholic fatty liver disease: practice Guideline by the American Association for the Study of Liver Diseases, American College of Gastroenterology, and the American Gastroenterological Association. Hepatology 2012;55:2005–2023.

19 Wieckowska A, McCullough AJ, Feldstein AE: Noninvasive diagnosis and monitoring of nonalcoholic steatohepatitis: present and future. Hepatology 2007;46:582–589.

20 Kashyap SR, Diab DL, Baker AR, Yerian L, Bajaj H, Gray-McGuire C, et al: Triglyceride levels and not adipokine concentrations are closely related to severity of nonalcoholic fatty liver disease in an obesity surgery cohort. Obesity (Silver Spring) 2009;17:1696–1701.

21 Campos GM, Bambha K, Vittinghoff E, Rabl C, Posselt AM, Ciovica R, et al: A clinical scoring system for predicting nonalcoholic steatohepatitis in morbidly obese patients. Hepatology 2008;47:1916–1923.

22 Sumida Y, Yoneda M, Hyogo H, Yamaguchi K, Ono M, Fujii H, et al: A simple clinical scoring system using ferritin, fasting insulin, and type IV collagen 7S for predicting steatohepatitis in nonalcoholic fatty liver disease. J Gastroenterol 2011;46:257–268.

23 Hashimoto E, Yatsuji S, Kaneda H, Yoshioka Y, Taniai M, Tokushige K, et al: The characteristics and natural history of Japanese patients with nonalcoholic fatty liver disease. Hepatol Res 2005;33:72–76.

24 Fitzpatrick E, Mitry RR, Quaglia A, Hussain MJ, DeBruyne R, Dhawan A: Serum levels of CK18 M30 and leptin are useful predictors of steatohepatitis and fibrosis in paediatric NAFLD. J Pediatr Gastroenterol Nutr 2010; 51:500–506.

25 Fealy CE, Haus JM, Solomon TP, Pagadala M, Flask CA, McCullough AJ, et al: Short-term exercise reduces markers of hepatocyte apoptosis in nonalcoholic fatty liver disease. J Appl Physiol (1985) 2012;113:1–6.

26 Vos MB, Barve S, Joshi-Barve S, Carew JD, Whitington PF, McClain CJ: Cytokeratin 18, a marker of cell death, is increased in children with suspected nonalcoholic fatty liver disease. J Pediatr Gastroenterol Nutr 2008;47: 481–485.

27 Haukeland JW, Damås JK, Konopski Z, Løberg EM, Haaland T, Goverud I, et al: Systemic inflammation in nonalcoholic fatty liver disease is characterized by elevated levels of CCL2. J Hepatol 2006;44:1167–1174.

28 Shimada M, Kawahara H, Ozaki K, Fukura M, Yano H, Tsuchishima M, et al: Usefulness of a combined evaluation of the serum adiponectin level, HOMA-IR, and serum type IV collagen 7S level to predict the early stage of nonalcoholic steatohepatitis. Am J Gastroenterol 2007;102:1931–1938.

29 Cao W, Zhao C, Shen C, Wang Y: Cytokeratin 18, alanine aminotransferase, platelets and triglycerides predict the presence of nonalcoholic steatohepatitis. PLoS One 2013;8:1–8.

Original Article

Digestive Diseases

Dig Dis 2015;33:721–727
DOI: 10.1159/000439078

Characteristics of Hypovascular versus Hypervascular Well-Differentiated Hepatocellular Carcinoma Smaller Than 2 cm – Focus on Tumor Size, Markers and Imaging Detectability

Kayo Sugimoto[a, c] Soo Ryang Kim[b] Susumu Imoto[b] Madoka Tohyama[b] Soo Ki Kim[e] Toshiyuki Matsuoka[f] Yoshihiko Yano[d] Masatoshi Kudo[g] Yoshitake Hayashi[c]

[a]Department of Pharmacy and [b]Department of Gastroenterology, Kobe Asahi Hospital, Kobe, [c]Division of Molecular Medicine and Medical Genetics and [d]Division of Center Infectious Diseases, Department of Pathology, Kobe University Graduate School of Medicine, Kobe, [e]Department of Gastroenterology and Hepatology, Kyoto University, Kyoto, [f]Department of Radiology, Osaka City University Medical School, Osaka, [g]Department of Gastroenterology and Hepatology, Kinki University School of Medicine, Osaka-Sayama, Osaka, Japan

Key Words

Hypovascular well-differentiated HCC · Early HCC · Imaging detectability · Gd-EOB-DTPA MRI · Hepatobiliary phase · International working group · Arterioportal angiography

Abstract

Objectives: The characteristics of hypovascular and hypervascular well-differentiated hepatocellular carcinomas (HCCs) were compared in terms of tumor size, tumor markers and detectability by imaging modalities. ***Methods:*** Well-differentiated HCC nodules that are smaller than 2 cm (n = 27) were evaluated in 27 patients using histopathology and divided into 2 groups: hypovascular (n = 10) and hypervascular (n = 17). The diagnostic sensitivity of imaging modalities was then evaluated for efficiency in disclosing tumor size and tumor markers in the 2 types. ***Results:*** No difference was observed in tumor size and tumor markers between the 2 types; however, the sensitivity of contrast-enhanced CT, contrast-enhanced ultrasonography and arterioportal angiography was significantly different between the 2 types, whereas that by Gadolinium-ethoxybenzyl-diethylenetriamine pentaacetic acid enhanced magnetic resonance imaging (Gd-EOB-DTPA MRI) demonstrated no difference. ***Conclusion:*** Hypovascular HCC could be diagnosed by Gd-EOB-DTPA MRI in the hepatobiliary phase.

Introduction

Recent studies support the division of small hepatocellular carcinoma (HCC) into 2 clinicopathological categories termed early HCC and progressed HCC; the former has a vaguely nodular appearance and is well-differentiated, whereas the latter has a distinctly nodular pattern and is mostly moderately differentiated, often with evidence of microvascular invasion [1, 2].

The characteristic imaging appearance of progressed HCC, a hypervascular lesion that shows washout in the portal venous phase, is also typical in small HCCs of the distinctly nodular type and in most moderately differentiated and some well-differentiated small HCCs [3–7]. Most early HCCs are hypovascular lesions. Hypovascular well-differentiated HCC is considered an early HCC, as proposed by the International Working Group [8].

KARGER 125

E-Mail karger@karger.com
www.karger.com/ddi

Soo Ryang Kim, MD
Department of Gastroenterology
Kobe Asahi Hospital
3-5-25 Bououji-cho, Nagata-ku, Kobe, 653-0801 (Japan)
E-Mail asahi-hp@arion.ocn.ne.jp

These classic images are explained by the anatomic features of the lesions. Hypovascularity, hypervascularity and isovascularity are understood to mean signal intensity in the arterial phase of contrast-enhanced imaging relative to the non-tumorous liver. Hypervascularity is related to the development of unpaired arteries, the absence of portal vein supply and the distinctly nodular growth [9].

From the view point of vascularity, 2 well-differentiated HCCs are categorized as hypovascular HCC and hypervascular HCC; however, they cannot be differentiated by routine ultrasonography (US) patterns.

Comparison of tumor size, tumor markers and imaging detectability in hypovascular and hypervascular HCCs remains to be clarified.

Here, to characterize hypovascular well-differentiated HCC, tumor size, tumor markers and imaging detectability were evaluated and compared with those of hypervascular well-differentiated HCCs.

Table 1. Patient baseline characteristics in hypovascular and hypervascular HCCs

	Hypovascular HCC (n = 10)	Hypervascular HCC (n = 17)
Age, years, mean ± SD	71.0±6.88	71.8±5.61
Range	60–81	59–81
Sex, male/female	5/5	8/9
Cause, n		
HBV	1	0
HCV	8	11
Non-HBV/HCV	0	1
Alcohol	1	5

Materials and Methods

Patients

From April 2008 to December 2009, a total of 27 nodules that were smaller than 2 cm diagnosed as well-differentiated HCC by histopathological analysis in 27 patients (13 men and 14 women, 71.5 ± 5.99 years) with liver cirrhosis related to the hepatitis B virus (HBV; n = 1), hepatitis C virus (HCV; n = 19), alcohol (n = 6) and non-HBV/HCV (n = 1) were retrospectively examined (table 1). The study was approved by the Ethics Committee at Kobe Asahi Hospital.

Assay of Serum Levels of Alpha-Fetoprotein and PIVKA II

Serum alpha-fetoprotein (AFP) concentrations were determined with a commercially available electrochemiluminescence immunoassay kit (Elecsys AFP immunoassay, Roche, Mannheim, Germany). Serum prothrombin induced by vitamin K absence II (PIVKA II) level was measured by revised enzyme immunoassay (Eitest PIVKA II; Eisai, Tokyo, Japan).

Contrast-Enhanced CT

Contrast-enhanced CT (CECT) was performed with the use of helical CT (Siemens, Germany) with pre- and post-contrast triple-phase (arterial, portal, venous and equilibrium phases) scans, after the injection of 120 ml of non-ionic contrast medium at 3 ml/s; the scans were carried out in a craniocaudal direction with 5 mm collimation in the other phases. Acquisition of the arterial and equilibrium phases was automatically started at 30 and 180 s, respectively, after the intravenous injection.

Contrast-Enhanced US

US was carried out with an SSA-660A system (Toshiba Medical Systems, Tochigi, Japan). The vascular findings on phase-inversion harmonic US were shown as tumor vessel flow in the early vascular phase about 15–40 s after the injection of Sonazoid (GE HealthCare, Piscataway, N.J., USA). Real-time replenishing images were acquired during the vascular phase (<2 min after the injection) by release-burst imaging. Images of liver parenchyma were acquired in the post-vascular Kupffer phase, at least 10 min after the intravenous injection of Sonazoid. Hepatic malignances were visualized as defects in the post-vascular phase. An additional contrast agent was injected to confirm tumor vessel flow in the defect, a technique known as defect reperfusion imaging [10].

Gadolinium-Ethoxybenzyl-Diethylenetriamine Pentaacetic Acid Enhanced MRI

Images by MRI scans (Philips, The Netherlands) were obtained using the 1.0-Tesla superconducting system (Gyroscan 10T-NT, Philips, The Netherlands). Enhanced MRI was used to acquire coronal images by the gradient-echo technique (fixed-field gradient) at 150/3.5 ms TR/TE, 80° flip angle and a 168 × 256 matrix. In each sequence, the respiration suspension time was 20–30 s. Gadolinium-ethoxybenzyl-diethylenetriamine pentaacetic acid enhanced (Gd-EOB-DTPA) MRI (Primovist; Bayer HealthCare, Osaka, Japan) at a dose of 0.025 mmol/kg body weight was injected intravenously as a rapid bolus at 2 ml/s. Dynamic contrast-enhanced MRI was initiated at 30 and 70 s, 2–3 and 20 min after the start of the bolus injection to acquire multiphasic (arterial, portal, late and hepatobiliary) images.

CT Arterioportal Angiography (CTA and CTAP)

CT during Arteriography (CTA). At angiography, 45 ml of diluted contrast medium was injected through a catheter at 2 ml/s into the common hepatic artery. The whole liver was then scanned at intervals of 5–10 mm.

CT during Arterial Portography (CTAP). At angiography, 115 ml of diluted contrast medium was injected through a catheter at 2 ml/s into the superior mesenteric artery, according to the scanning time of the entire liver, using a power injector during sequential scanning, with incremental changes in the position of the table. Infusion of contrast material was initiated 20 s before CTAP. The whole liver was then scanned at intervals of 5–10 mm.

US-Guided Biopsy

US-guided biopsy was carried out with the use of a 21-gauge Majima needle (Top, Japan). The diagnosis of HCC was made by K.S. and Y.H. using the same specimen.

Histological Diagnosis

Specimens were routinely processed and stained with hematoxylin and eosin and by the Masson trichromatic method. The diagnosis of HCC was made according to the criteria of the International Working Party [8].

Imaging Patterns for Conclusive Diagnosis of HCC by the 4 Modalities

The following patterns disclosed by the 4 imaging modalities were conclusive diagnosis of HCC: (1) CECT, hypervascularity in the arterial phase and washout in the equilibrium phase; (2) Sonazoid contrast-enhanced ultrasonography (CEUS), hypervascularity in the early vascular phase and defect in the Kupffer phase; (3) Gd-EOB-DTPA MRI, hypervascularity in the arterial phase and/or defect in the hepatobiliary phase and (4) CT arterioportal angiography, hypervascularity by CTA and/or perfusion defect by CTAP (table 2).

Imaging Studies

To minimize differences in the results between the operators, imaging studies were carried out and reviewed by M.K. and T.M. using the same examination protocol.

Statistical Analysis

The comparisons of sensitivity of tumor size, tumor markers and imaging detectability between hypovascular and hypervascular HCCs were assessed by univariate analysis using the Mann-Whitney U test and χ^2 test. Variables with a p value of <0.05 were considered statistically significant. All statistical analyses were carried out with EXCEL multivariate statistical analysis software, version 6.0 (ESUMI Inc., Toyo, Japan).

Table 2. Imaging patterns for conclusive diagnosis of HCC by the 4 modalities

Modality	Imaging pattern
CECT	Hypervascularity in the arterial phase and washout in the equilibrium phase
CEUS	Hypervascularity in the early vascular phase and defect in the Kupffer phase
Gd-EOB-DTPA MRI	Hypervascularity in the arterial phase and/or defect in the hepatobiliary phase
CTA and CTAP	Hypervascularity by CTA and/or perfusion defect by CTAP

Table 3. Tumor size and tumor marker in hypovascular and hypervascular HCCs

	Hypovascular HCC (n = 10)	Hypervascular HCC (n = 17)	p value
Tumor size, mm	11.9±2.6	12.0±3.7	0.940
AFP, ng/ml	7.7±5.4	53.7±118.9	0.236
PIVKA II, mAU/ml	35.6±43.8	52.3±96.8	0.613

Values are shown as means ± SD.

Table 4. The sensitivity of imaging in hypovascular and hypervascular HCCs

	Hypovascular HCC (n = 10)	Hypervascular HCC (n = 17)	p value
CEUS	0	8	0.011
CECT	0	7	0.022
Gd-EOB DTPA MRI	9	14	0.523
CTA and CTAP	6	17	0.012

Values are shown as number of persons.

Results

Among the 27 well-differentiated HCC nodules, 10 were categorized as hypovascular and 17 as hypervascular, with no difference in size between the 2 types (hypovascular HCC: 11.9 ± 2.6 mm, hypervascular HCC: 12.0 ± 3.7 mm). The average AFP value was 7.7 ± 5.4 ng/ml for hypovascular HCC and 53.7 ± 118.9 ng/ml for hypervascular HCC. The average PIVKA II was 35.6 ± 43.8 mAU/ml for hypovascular HCC and 52.3 ± 98.6 mAU/ml for hypervascular HCC. Tumor markers showed no difference between the 2 types (AFP: p = 0.236, PIVKA II: p = 0.613; table 3).

Imaging sensitivity for hypovascular HCC was 0% (0 of 10) by CECT, 0% (0 of 10) by CEUS, 90% (9 of 10) by Gd-EOB-DTPA MRI and 60% (6 of 10) by CT arterioportal angiography. For hypervascular HCC, the respective sensitivity was 41% (7 of 17) by CECT, 47% (8 of 17) by CEUS, 82% (14 of 17) by Gd-EOB-DTPA MRI and 100% (17 of 17) by CT arterioportal angiography. A difference was observed in the sensitivity by CECT (p = 0.022), CEUS (p = 0.011) and CT arterioportal angiography (p = 0.012) between the 2 types of HCCs; no difference was observed in the sensitivity by Gd-EOB-DTPA MRI (p = 0.523; table 4).

Representative Cases

Case No. 1. Hypervascular well-differentiated HCC was detected by CT arterioportal angiography (CTA and CTAP) in a 63-year-old woman with alcohol-related liver cirrhosis (AFP 5.2 ng/ml, PIVKA II 34 mAU/ml). US revealed a 15 mm hypoechoic nodule in segment 8 (fig. 1a).

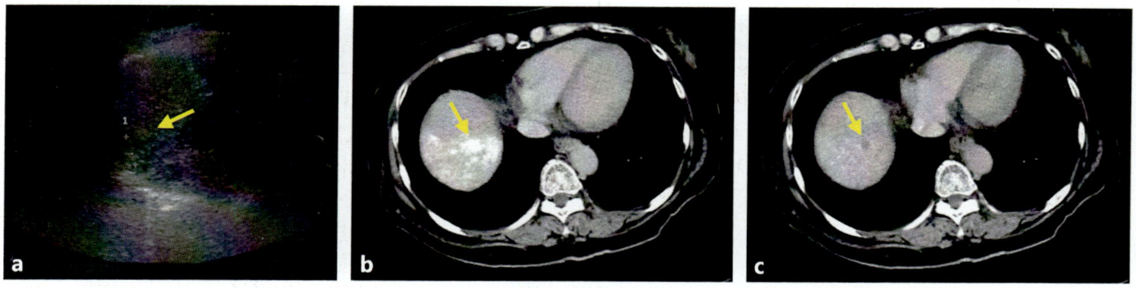

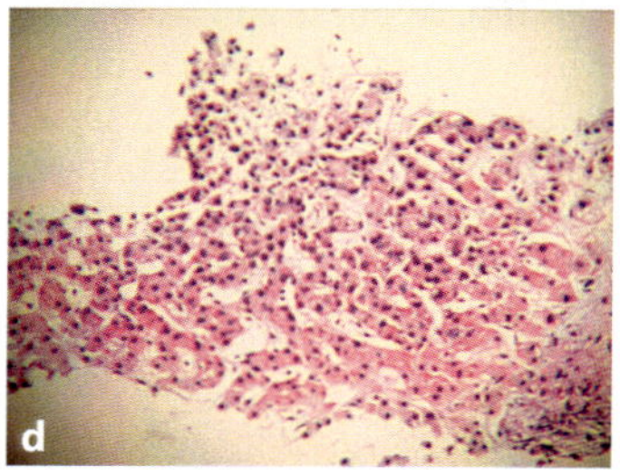

Fig. 1. Case No. 1: Hypervascular well-differentiated HCC detected by CT arterioportal angiography. Imaging and histological findings of the nodule in segment 8. **a** US reveals a 15-mm hypoechoic nodule (arrow); **b**, **c** CTA reveals a hypervascular nodule (**b**) and CTAP (**c**) reveals a perfusion defect (arrow); **d** Histological finding of US-guided biopsy HE stained well-differentiated HCC characterized by moderate hypercellularity with slight cell atypia and eosinophilia are observed.

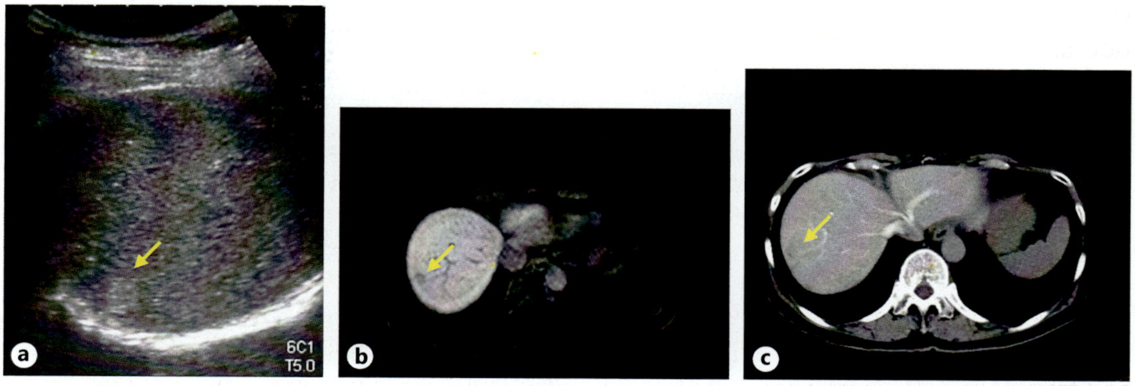

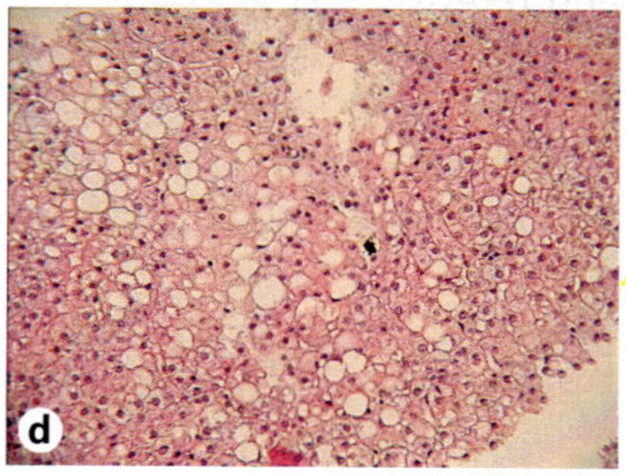

Fig. 2. Case No. 2: Hypovascular well-differentiated HCC detected by Gd-EOB-DTPA MRI and CTAP. Imaging and histological findings of the nodule in segment 8. **a** US reveals a 14-mm hyperechoic nodule in segment 8 (arrow); **b** Gd-EOB-DTPA MRI reveals a defect in the hepatobiliary phase (arrow); **c** CTAP reveals a perfusion defect (arrow); **d** HE staining. Slight hypercellularity with cell atypia and diffuse fatty change.

CEUS revealed no hypervascularity in the early phase and no defect in the Kupffer phase. CECT revealed no hypervascularity in the early phase and no washout in the equilibrium phase. Gd-EOB-DTPA MRI revealed no hypervascularity in the arterial phase and no defect in the hepatobiliary phase. CTA revealed a hypervascular nodule (fig. 1b) and CTAP revealed a perfusion defect (fig. 1c). US-guided biopsy revealed well-differentiated HCC characterized by moderate hypercellularity with slight cell atypia and eosinophilia (fig. 1d).

Case No. 2. Hypovascular well-differentiated HCC was detected by Gd-EOB-DTPA MRI and CT arterioportal angiography (CTAP) in a 68-year-old woman with chronic HCV infection (AFP 11.0 ng/ml, PIVKA II 14 mAU/ml). US revealed a 14 mm hyperechoic nodule in segment 8 (fig. 2a). CEUS revealed no hypovascularity in the early phase and no defect in the Kupffer phase. CECT revealed no hypervascularity in the early phase and no washout in the equilibrium phase. Gd-EOB-DTPA MRI revealed no hypervascularity in the arterial phase but disclosed a defect in the hepatobiliary phase (fig. 2b). CTA revealed no enhanced lesion, but CTAP revealed a perfusion defect (fig. 2c). Histological analysis of a US-guided biopsy revealed well-differentiated HCC characterized by slight hypercellularity with cell atypia and diffuse fatty change (fig. 2d).

Discussion

Recently clinicians have been able to conduct CTA, thereby acquiring data on lesions and intra-nodular blood flow simultaneously [11, 12].

Moreover, development of newly introduced diagnostic imaging techniques, Sonazoid CEUS and Gd-EOB-DTPA MRI has provided higher degrees of detectability for small HCC.

The status of imaging studies in the diagnosis of HCCs that are smaller than 2 cm has changed with the introduction of new contrast agents used in US and MRI. First, Sonazoid was exclusively approved in Japan in 2007 as a second-generation US contrast agent; Kudo et al. [10, 13, 14] have recently developed defect reperfusion imaging (featuring the properties of very stable Kupffer phase images and real-time fine blood flow images obtained with Sonazoid) for typical HCC, which is depicted by CT but not by B-mode scanning. The method is a breakthrough for accurate localization and treatment guidance [10]: dramatic resolution of many limitations in the diagnosis and treatment of HCC, such as detection of small HCCs [15], evaluation of treatment response [16] and needle insertion guidance; additionally, detection is even more sensitive than with multidetector CT [15].

Second, Gd-EOB-DTPA, a new liver-specific contrast agent used in MRI [17–19], was approved in Japan in 2008; this newly introduced agent is a hepatocyte-specific MRI contrast medium with a different mechanism that utilizes neither dynamic nor Kupffer cell imaging. It is useful in cases that would be difficult to diagnose by techniques such as dynamic MRI or superparamagnetic iron oxide MRI. Typical HCC displays high intensity with Gd-EOB-DTPA in the arterial-dominant phase and low intensity in the portal-dominant phase and thereafter. Thus, the diagnosis of HCC can be made approximately 10–20 min after the injection of Gd-EOB-DTPA.

The improvement in these 2 imaging modalities with the use of the newly introduced contrast agents has provided higher sensitivity for the diagnosis of nodules that are smaller than 2 cm than with SonoVue CEUS and CECT [20] or with SonoVue CEUS and Gd-EOB-DTPA MRI [21].

The sensitivity of CECT, Sonazoid US, Gd-EOB-DTPA MRI and CT arterioportal angiography has been compared in the diagnosis of HCC in nodules that are smaller than 2 cm [22]. In a study of 34 moderately differentiated (n = 24) and well-differentiated HCC (n = 10) nodules, the overall sensitivity has been 53.9% by CECT, 67.6% by Sonazoid-enhanced US, 76.5% by Gd-EOB-DTPA MRI and 88.2% by CT arterioportal angiography. A significant difference has been observed in the sensitivity between CECT and CT arterioportal angiography, but not among Sonazoid-enhanced US, Gd-EOB-DTPA MRI and CT arterioportal angiography. The authors have concluded that changing the main diagnostic modality for HCCs that are smaller than 2 cm from CT arterioportal angiography to Sonazoid-enhanced US and Gd-EOB-DTPA MRI is recommended [23].

From the view point of vascularity, well-differentiated HCC can be categorized as hypervascular and hypovascular HCCs. The present study was carried out because, to date, the difference between these categories in terms of tumor size, tumor markers and imaging detectability has not been characterized.

The results demonstrated no difference between hypervascular and hypovascular HCCs in tumor size and tumor markers including AFP and PIVKA II [24] (table 4); in other words, they could not be differentiated through tumor size or tumor markers.

In the diagnosis of hypovascular HCC, CECT and CEUS were totally ineffective, Gd-EOB-DTPA MRI was markedly effective and arterioportal angiography was moderately effective (table 3).

Histopathological findings have demonstrated that early HCC tumors are vaguely nodular and are characterized by various combinations of the following major features [25–27]: (1) increased cell density of more than 2 times that of the surrounding tissue, with an increased nuclear/cytoplasm ratio and an irregularly thin-trabecular pattern, (2) a varying number of portal tracts within the nodule (intra-tumoral portal tracts), (3) a pseudoglandular pattern, (4) diffuse fatty change and (5) a varying number of unpaired arteries.

Although most hypervascular and hypovascular well-differentiated HCCs (like representative cases 1 and 2) were characterized by the above major histological features, stromal invasion, described by the International Consensus Group for Hepatocellular Neoplasia as helpful in differentiating early HCC from high-grade dysplastic nodules [9], is invasion into portal tracks of septal stroma within a hepatocellular nodule and is confirmed by Victoria blue staining.

Dig Dis 2015;33:721–727
DOI: 10.1159/000439078

Stromal invasion, which may be difficult to identify in early HCC because tumor cells show little or no cytologic atypia, is often focal; its identification is still more difficult when dealing with biopsied liver tissue in which only limited portions of nodules are sampled. CK7 immunostaining is useful in identifying stromal invasion. Ductular reaction, confirmed by CK7 immunostaining, is frequently found in non-cancerous hepatocellular nodular lesions, whereas it is less frequently found in HCCs with true stromal invasion [23].

Early HCC takes longer to recur and has a higher 5-year survival rate than progressed HCC [28]. The prognosis of early HCC is considered good because of the absence of portal invasion and daughter nodules [29].

Thus, the diagnosis of hypovascular well-differentiated HCC will gain increasing importance in the management of HCC.

In conclusion, in view of the invasiveness of CT arterioportal angiography, the imaging algorithm focused on Gd-EOB-DTPA MRI in the hepatobiliary phase for the diagnosis of hypovascular HCC is routinely used in clinical settings in Japan [4, 19]. Here, we strongly recommend the use of this imaging modality in other countries where HCC is endemic.

Acknowledgment

We are indebted to Ms. Mika Matsui for assistance in the preparation of this manuscript.

Disclosure Statement

The authors declare that they have no financial conflict of interest.

References

1 Kojiro M, Nakashima O: Histopathologic evaluation of hepatocellular carcinoma with special reference to small early stage tumors. Semin Liver Dis 1999;19:287–296.
2 Kudo M: Early hepatocellular carcinoma: definition and diagnosis. Liver Cancer 2013;2:69–72.
3 Murakami T, Tsurusaki M: Hypervascular benign and malignant liver tumors that require differentiation from hepatocellular carcinoma: key points of imaging diagnosis. Liver Cancer 2014;3:85–96.
4 Kudo M, Matsui O, Izumi N, Iijima H, Kadoya M, Imai Y, Okusaka T, Miyayama S, Tsuchiya K, Ueshima K, Hiraoka A, Ikeda M, Ogasawara S, Yamashita T, Minami T, Yamakado K; Liver Cancer Study Group of Japan: JSH consensus-based clinical practice guidelines for the management of hepatocellular carcinoma: 2014 update by the liver cancer study group of Japan. Liver Cancer 2014;3:458–468.
5 Kudo M: Surveillance, diagnosis, treatment, and outcome of liver cancer in Japan. Liver Cancer 2015;4:39–50.
6 Kudo M: Clinical practice guidelines for hepatocellular carcinoma differ between Japan, United States, and Europe. Liver Cancer 2015;4:85–95.
7 Hsu C, Chen BB, Chen CH, Ho MC, Cheng JC, Kokudo N, Murakami T, Yeo W, Seong J, Jia JD, Han KH, Cheng AL: Consensus development from the 5th Asia-Pacific primary liver cancer expert meeting (APPLE 2014). Liver Cancer 2015;4:96–105.
8 International Working Party: Terminology of nodular hepatocellular lesions. Hepatology 1995;22:983–993.
9 International Consensus Group for Hepatocellular Neoplasia: Pathologic diagnosis of early hepatocellular carcinoma: a report of the international consensus group for hepatocellular neoplasia. Hepatology 2009;49:658–664.
10 Kudo M, Hatanaka K, Chung H, Minami Y, Maekawa K: A proposal of novel treatment-assist technique for hepatocellular carcinoma in the Sonazoid-enhanced ultrasonography: value of defect re-perfusion imaging. Kanzo 2007;48:299–301.
11 Hayashi M, Matsui O, Ueda K, Kawamori Y, Gabata T, Kadoya M: Progression to hypervascular hepatocellular carcinoma: correlation with intranodular blood supply evaluated with CT during intraarterial injection of contrast material. Radiology 2002;225:143–149.
12 Tajima T, Honda H, Taguchi K, Asayama Y, Kuroiwa T, Yoshimitsu K, Irie H, Aibe H, Shimada M, Masuda K: Sequential hemodynamic change in hepatocellular carcinoma and dysplastic nodules: CT angiography and pathologic correlation. AJR Am J Roentgenol 2002;178:885–897.
13 Kudo M, Hatanaka K, Maekawa K: Defect reperfusion imaging, a newly developed novel technology using Sonazoid in the treatment of hepatocellular carcinoma. J Med Ultrasound 2008;16:169–175.
14 Kudo M, Hatanaka K, Maekawa K: Sonazoid-enhanced ultrasound in the diagnosis and treatment of hepatic tumors. J Med Ultrasound 2008;16:130–139.
15 Hatanaka K, Kudo M, Minami Y, Maekawa K: Sonazoid-enhanced ultrasonography for diagnosis of hepatic malignancies: comparison with contrast-enhanced CT. Oncology 2008;75(suppl 1):42–47.
16 Xia Y, Kudo M, Minami Y, Hatanaka K, Ueshima K, Chung H, Hagiwara S, Inoue T, Ishikawa E, Kitai S, Takahashi S, Tatsumi C, Ueda T, Hayaishi S, Maekawa K: Response evaluation of transcatheter arterial chemoembolization in hepatocellular carcinomas: the usefulness of Sonazoid-enhanced harmonic sonography. Oncology 2008;75(suppl 1):99–105.
17 Lee JM, Yoon JH, Joo I, Woo HS: Recent advances in CT and MR imaging for evaluation of hepatocellular carcinoma. Liver Cancer 2012;1:22–40.
18 Ricke J, Seidensticker M, Mohnike K: Noninvasive diagnosis of hepatocellular carcinoma in cirrhotic liver: current guidelines and future prospects for radiological imaging. Liver Cancer 2012;1:51–58.
19 Ichikawa T, Sano K, Morisaka H: Diagnosis of pathologically early HCC with EOB-MRI: experiences and current consensus. Liver Cancer 2014;3:97–107.
20 Bolondi L, Gaiani S, Celli N, Golfieri R, Grigioni WF, Leoni S, Venturi AM, Piscaglia F: Characterization of small nodules in cirrhosis by assessment of vascularity: the problem of hypovascular hepatocellular carcinoma. Hepatology 2005;42:27–34.
21 Forner A, Vilana R, Ayuso C, Bianchi L, Solé M, Ayuso JR, Boix L, Sala M, Varela M, Llovet JM, Brú C, Bruix J: Diagnosis of hepatic nodules 20 mm or smaller in cirrhosis: prospective validation of the noninvasive diagnostic criteria for hepatocellular carcinoma. Hepatology 2008;47:97–104.

22 Mita K, Kim SR, Kudo M, Imoto S, Nakajima T, Ando K, Fukuda K, Matsuoka T, Maekawa Y, Hayashi Y: Diagnostic sensitivity of imaging modalities for hepatocellular carcinoma smaller than 2 cm. World J Gastroenterol 2010;16:4187–4192.
23 Kobayashi S, Kim SR, Imoto S, Ando K, Hirakawa M, Saito J, Fukuda K, Otono Y, Sakaki M, Tsuchida S, Kim SK, Hayashi Y, Nakano M, Kudo M: Histopathological diagnosis of early HCC through biopsy: efficacy of victoria blue and cytokeratin 7 staining. Dig Dis 2012; 30:574–579.
24 Toyoda H, Kumada T, Tada T, Sone Y, Kaneoka Y, Maeda A: Tumor markers for hepatocellular carcinoma: simple and significant predictors of outcome in patients with HCC. Liver Cancer 2015;4:126–136.
25 Hytiroglou P: Morphological changes of early human hepatocarcinogenesis. Semin Liver Dis 2004;24:65–75.
26 Kojiro M: Pathology of Hepatocellular Carcinoma. Oxford, Blackwell Publishing, 2006.
27 Hytiroglou P, Park YN, Krinsky G, Theise ND: Hepatic precancerous lesions and small hepatocellular carcinoma. Gastroenterol Clin North Am 2007;36:867–887.
28 Takayama T, Makuuchi M, Hirohashi S, Sakamoto M, Yamamoto J, Shimada K, Kosuge T, Okada S, Takayasu K, Yamasaki S: Early hepatocellular carcinoma as an entity with a high rate of surgical cure. Hepatology 1998;28:1241–1246.
29 Nakashima O, Sugihara S, Kage M, Kojiro M: Pathomorphologic characteristics of small hepatocellular carcinoma: a special reference to small hepatocellular carcinoma with indistinct margins. Hepatology 1995;22:101–105.

Original Article

Digestive Diseases

Dig Dis 2015;33:728–734
DOI: 10.1159/000439079

Real-Life Clinical Practice with Sorafenib in Advanced Hepatocellular Carcinoma: A Single-Center Experience Second Analysis

Tadaaki Arizumi Kazuomi Ueshima Mina Iwanishi Hirokazu Chishina Masashi Kono Masahiro Takita Satoshi Kitai Tatsuo Inoue Norihisa Yada Satoru Hagiwara Hiroshi Ida Yasunori Minami Toshiharu Sakurai Naoshi Nishida Masayuki Kitano Masatoshi Kudo

Department of Gastroenterology and Hepatology, Kinki University School of Medicine, Osaka-Sayama, Osaka, Japan

Key Words

Sorafenib · Hepatocellular carcinoma · Adverse events · RECICL

Abstract

Objectives: Sorafenib has become a standard therapy for advanced hepatocellular carcinoma following the demonstration of significant increase in progression-free survival as well as overall survival (OS) in the 2-phase III trials. We examined efficacy and adverse events (AEs) in patients treated with sorafenib over a 6-year period since approval in Japan. ***Methods:*** Two hundred and forty-one patients treated with sorafenib at the Kinki University Hospital were retrospectively analyzed clinically for the factors related to survival periods, tumor response evaluated by the Response Evaluation Criteria In Cancer of the Liver (RECICL) and AEs. ***Results:*** OS was 14.3 months. According to the RECICL, the objective response and disease control rates were 18.6% (43 of 241) and 61.1% (137 of 241), respectively. AEs were seen in 77.3% (187 of 241), with Grade 3 or higher in 23.6% (57 of 241). The most frequent AE was hand-foot skin reaction in 109 patients (45.0%), and 28 patients (11.8%) showed Grade 3 or higher. Significant factors contributing to the OS were treatment duration ($p = 0.0204$), up-to-7 criteria ($p = 0.0400$), increase of Child-Pugh score ($p = 0.0008$) and tumor response determined by the RECICL ($p = 0.0007$). ***Conclusion:*** Based on the analysis, using many cases at a single center, we concluded that continuation of treatment with sorafenib for ≥90 days without decrease of liver function was critical if tumor response was determined as stable disease or higher.

Introduction

Hepatocellular carcinoma (HCC) is the fifth most common cancer in the world, and the incidence is increasing worldwide [1]. Because most patients are diagnosed with advanced disease stages, only 30% of patients receive potentially curative therapies, such as surgical resection [2–4], transplantation [5–8] or percutaneous ablation [9–13]. A majority of patients with unresectable HCC usually undergo palliative treatments, such as transarterial chemoembolization (TACE) [14–16], hepatic arterial infusion chemotherapy (HAIC) [17] and system-

Masatoshi Kudo, MD, PhD
Department of Gastroenterology and Hepatology
Kinki University School of Medicine
377-2 Ohno-Higashi, Osaka-Sayama, Osaka 589-8511 (Japan)
E-Mail m-kudo@med.kindai.ac.jp

ic chemotherapy, including therapy using molecular targeted agents [17–20].

Sorafenib is currently the standard systemic therapeutic agent approved for treatment of advanced HCC in patients with well-preserved liver function (Child-Pugh class A), within Barcelona Clinic Liver Cancer (BCLC) stage C, and showing progressive disease (PD) after locoregional therapy [17, 21–23]. Treatment using sorafenib is recommended based on the efficacy and safety reported by the 2 global randomized controlled trials: the Sorafenib HCC Assessment Randomized Protocol (SHARP) and the Asia-Pacific trials [24, 25]. The efficacy and safety of sorafenib in clinical practice have been addressed by additional field practice experiences, such as the Global Investigation of Therapeutic Decisions in HCC and of Its Treatment with Sorafenib (GIDEON) study [26, 27]. In Japan, sorafenib has been administered based on the consensus-based treatment algorithm for HCC proposed by the Japan Society of Hepatology [28]. Sorafenib is also recommended if TACE [14, 29, 30] and HAIC are not applicable but patients still carry a preserved liver function with Child-Pugh class A. In a previous study, we reported that the duration of administration was a significant prognostic factor for sorafenib treatment. A blood chemical test related to liver functions, such as serum levels of bilirubin as well as the tumor markers alpha-fetoprotein (AFP) and des-gamma carboxyprothrombin (DCP), could also be a marker predicting an overall survival (OS) [31–34]. In the current study, we retrospectively investigated 356 HCC patients treated with sorafenib at the Kinki University Hospital to elucidate the efficacy of sorafenib treatment and the clinical outcomes.

Materials and Methods

Patients

Between May 2009 and April 2015, 356 patients with HCC were treated with sorafenib at the Kinki University Hospital. Among these patients, 241 patients met the inclusion criteria listed below and were enrolled in the present study. The diagnosis of HCC was made by histological or radiologic findings using contrast-enhanced CT and/or dynamic MRI. Information regarding clinicopathological variables including demographic characteristics complete blood count, albumin, AFP, DCP, alanine aminotransferase (ALT), alkaline phosphatase (ALP), tumor stage (including number of focal lesions and maximum diameter of lesions in a contrast-enhancing disease), up-to-7 criteria and BCLC prognostic score were collected prior to treatment [35].

The inclusion criteria were as follows: (1) HCC diagnosed by histological examination or typical radiological findings (early enhancement followed by late washout on contrast-enhanced CT or dynamic MRI) and HCC refractory to radiofrequency ablation and TACE based on the indications for sorafenib, (2) Eastern Cooperative Oncology Group performance status of 0 or 1 and (3) Child-Pugh class A or B liver function. The exclusion criteria were as follows: (1) concomitant antineoplastic treatment and (2) TACE or radiofrequency ablation performed within 3 months of initiation of sorafenib. Our institution did not require informed consent for the review of patient records and images for a retrospective study, such as this was.

Treatment Strategy Using Sorafenib

Sorafenib was administered orally at a dose of 400 mg, twice daily. The initial dose was reduced by each attending physician according to the clinical conditions such as body weight, age, Eastern Cooperative Oncology Group performance status and liver function. Dose reduction and interruption of sorafenib were allowed and depended on the type and severity of adverse events (AEs). Dose reduction and discontinuation were determined based on the information in the package inserts. We continued sorafenib administration until the appearance of either intolerable toxicity or definitive progression of HCC. All AEs were graded according to the National Cancer Institute Common Terminology Criteria for AEs version 4.0 (CTCAE v4.0).

Follow-Up

Clinical and laboratory assessments and radiological evaluation were performed monthly and at 4- to 12-week intervals, respectively. Radiological assessment was blinded to the evolution of the disease and the patient outcomes. The patients who died before the first imaging assessment were classified as having experienced progression. OS was measured from the date of sorafenib initiation until the date of death.

Response Evaluation Using the RECICL

The Response Evaluation Criteria In Cancer of the Liver (RECICL) requires 2-directional measurement of tumors showing arterial enhancement. Complete response (CR) was defined as either a 100% tumor necrotizing effect or a 100% reduction in tumor size accompanied by disappearance of all contrast enhancements at any phase. Partial response (PR) was defined as either a 50% or greater reduction in tumor necrosis or size as determined by the 2-directional measurement. PD was defined as either a 50% or greater increase in tumor size or the appearance of one or more new lesions. The RECICL defined stable disease (SD) as the absence of either PR or PD; objective response rate as the percentage of CR + PR among all cases and disease control rate as the percentage of cases showing CR, PR or SD [36].

Statistical Analysis

Survival curves were calculated using the Kaplan–Meier method with the primary end point of death for analysis of OS. Patients who did not meet the end point were censored at the time of the last follow-up visit. Comparison of survival rates among the groups was estimated using the log-rank test, and comparison of categorical variables was performed using the χ^2 test. For multiple comparisons, the Bonferroni correction was applied. A p value of <0.05 was considered statistically significant. All analyses were performed using the SAS statistical software version 8.2 (SAS Institute, Cary, N.C., USA), or the SPSS Medical Pack for Windows version 10.0 (SPSS, Inc., Chicago, Ill., USA).

Table 1. Patient characteristics

	Cases, n	%
Age, years		
Median (25–75%)	73 (66–77)*	
Gender		
Male	180	74.7
Female	61	25.3
ECOG PS		
0	225	93.4
1	16	6.6
Up-to-7 criteria		
Within	64	26.6
Beyond	177	73.4
Virus status†		
Hepatitis B virus	43	17.8
Hepatitis C virus	121	50.2
Virus negative	77	32.0
BCLC stage		
A	30	12.4
B	65	27.0
C	146	60.6
Initial dose of sorafenib, mg		
200	20	8.3
400	94	39.0
800	127	52.7
Duration of sorafenib, days		
Median (25–75%)	78 (28–239)*	
Biochemical analysis, median (25–75%)		
Alanine aminotransferases, IU/l	33 (22–57)*	
Alkaline phosphatase, IU/l	405.4 (303–598.8)*	
White blood cell count, /μl	4,900 (3,900–6,400)*	
Hemoglobin, g/dl	12.4 (11.1–13.5)*	
Platelet count, $\times 10^4$/dl	14.2 (9.5–20.5)*	
α-Fetoprotein, ng/dl	186 (14–4,243)*	
α-Fetoprotein L3, %	16.1 (0.6–49.3)*	
Des-γ carboxyprothrombin, mAU/dl	1,115.5 (78.5–9,884)*	

* Dispersion variables are shown as median values (25–75%).
† Cases testing positive for hepatitis B virus surface antigen were regarded as cases of hepatitis B virus-related HCC and cases testing positive for hepatitis C antibody were regarded as cases of hepatitis C virus-related HCC.

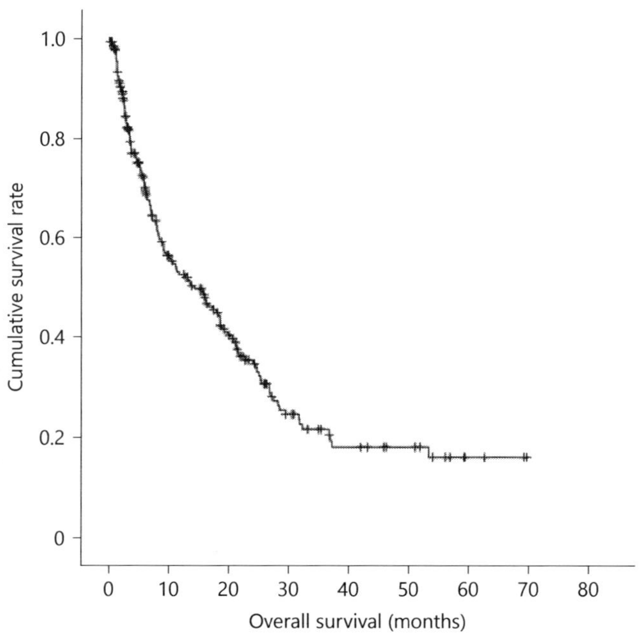

Fig. 1. OS of all patients treated with sorafenib. The Kaplan–Meier curves of the OS of the 241 patients who underwent treatment with sorafenib alone. Median survival time was 14.3 months (95% CI 9.3–18.6 months), and the 1- and 2-year survival rates were 52.5 and 34.6%, respectively.

Results

Baseline Characteristics

The baseline characteristics of the patients are summarized in table 1. The patients, predominantly men (74.7%), had a median age of 73 years. Two hundred twenty-five patients (93.4%) were asymptomatic, with a PS of 0. One hundred twenty-one patients (50.2%) tested positive for the anti-hepatitis C virus antibody, 43 patients (17.8%) were positive for the hepatitis B virus surface antigen and 77 patients (32.0%) were negative for both. Sixty-four patients (26.6%) met the up-to-7 criteria [37]. The initial sorafenib dose in this study ranged from 200 to 800 mg/day. An initial dose of 800 mg/day was administered in 127 patients (52.7%).

After a month of treatment with sorafenib, 106 patients experienced a continuous or transient increase in the Child-Pugh score, while 82 patients showed no change and 24 patients showed a decrease in the Child-Pugh score by least 1 point. Twenty-nine patients were not evaluated.

Prior treatment in the 203 cases included 60 resections, 116 local ablations, 164 cases of TACE, 34 cases of cytotoxic chemotherapy, 11 cases of radiation therapy and 29 cases of HAIC.

HCC Response to Sorafenib

The median OS of the entire cohort was 14.3 months (range 9.3–18.6 months). The 1- and 2-year survival rates were 52.5 and 34.6%, respectively (fig. 1). The numbers of patients with CR, PR, SD and PD were 7, 34, 94 and 86, respectively. The objective response rate and disease control rate as estimated by the RECICL were 18.6 and 61.1%, re-

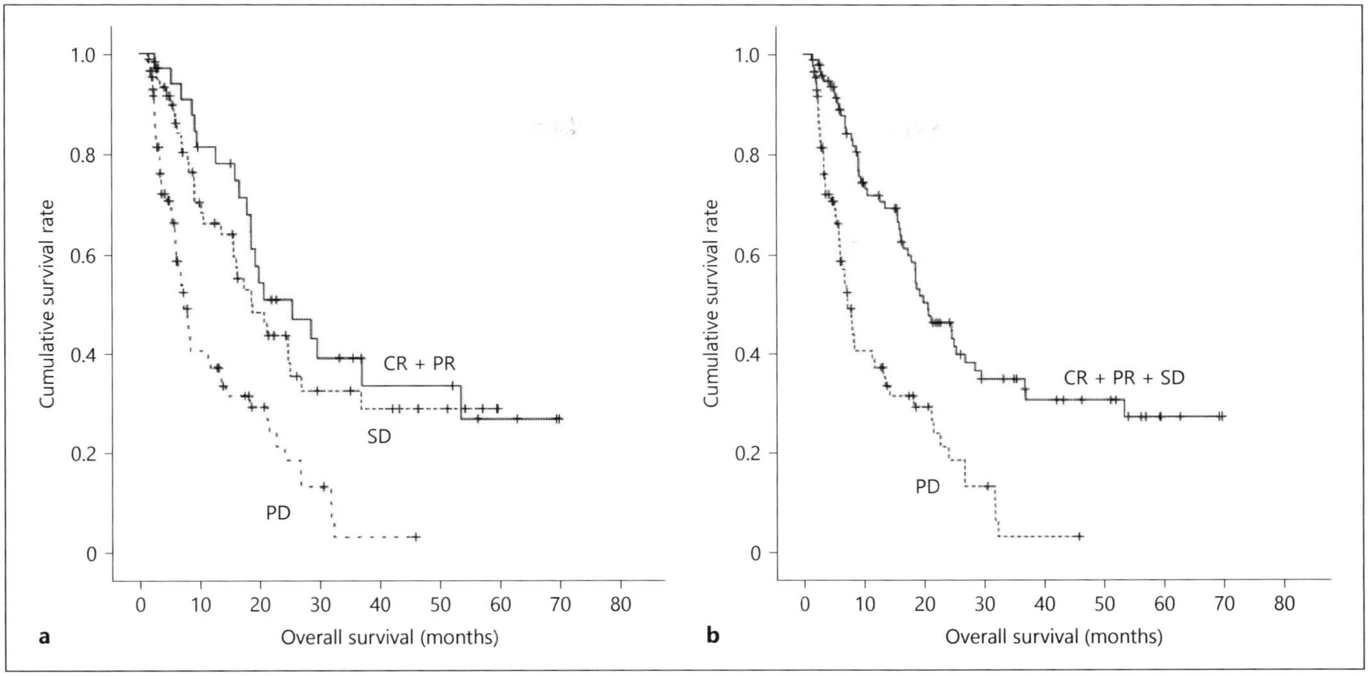

Fig. 2. The Kaplan–Meier curves of OS based on response to treatment as estimated by the RECICL. The Kaplan–Meier curves of the OS of the 221 patients based on response to sorafenib therapy as estimated by the RECICL. **a** The median OS of the patients classified as CR + PR, SD and PD, respectively, was 25.4, 18.8 and 7.3 months by the RECICL ($p < 0.0001$ by log-rank test). **b** The median OS of the patients classified as CR + PR + SD and PD, respectively, was 20.7 and 7.3 months by the RECICL ($p < 0.0001$ by log-rank test).

spectively. Twenty patients were not evaluated. We compared the OS among the CR + PR, SD and PD groups using the Kaplan–Meier estimates. The comparisons of the survival curves showed that the median OS was 25.4 months (95% CI 17.9–53.4 months) in the CR + PR group, 18.8 months (95% CI 13.6–25.1 months) in the SD group and 7.3 months (95% CI 6.0–11.8 months) in the PD group ($p < 0.001$; fig. 2a). Pairwise comparisons verified a significantly longer OS in the CR + PR group than in the PD group ($p < 0.001$ by the log-rank test). Similarly, OS was significantly longer in the SD group than in the PD group ($p = 0.001$). In contrast, no significant differences in OS were detected between the CR + PR and SD groups ($p = 0.392$). We also compared the OS between the CR + PR + SD group and the PD group using the Kaplan–Meier estimates. The comparisons of the survival curves showed that the median OS was 20.7 months (95% CI 16.7–26.9 months) in the CR + PR + SD group and 7.3 months (95% CI 6.0–11.8 months) in the PD group ($p < 0.001$; fig. 2b).

Prognostic Factors of HCC Patients Treated with Sorafenib

We analyzed the baseline patient characteristics to identify factors that affected OS after sorafenib therapy. Univariate analysis revealed statistically significant differences in OS for the following variables: treatment duration ($p < 0.0001$), up-to-7 criteria ($p < 0.0001$), portal invasion ($p < 0.0001$), extrahepatic spread ($p = 0.0018$), PS ($p = 0.0113$), albumin ($p = 0.0004$), total bilirubin ($p < 0.0001$), white blood cell count ($p = 0.0172$), platelet count ($p = 0.0335$), ALT ($p = 0.0136$), ALP ($p = 0.0163$), AFP ($p < 0.0001$), DCP ($p < 0.0001$), AFP-L3 ($p = 0.0131$), BCLC stage ($p = 0.0006$), Child-Pugh score increase ($p < 0.0001$) and response evaluation using the RECICL ($p < 0.0001$) at the initiation of sorafenib therapy (table 2). Multivariate analysis revealed statistically significant differences in OS for the following variables: treatment duration ($p = 0.0204$), up-to-7 criteria ($p = 0.0400$), Child-Pugh score increase ($p = 0.0008$) and response evaluation using the RECICL ($p = 0.0007$; table 3).

Drug-Related AEs of Sorafenib

The overall incidence of drug-related AEs of any grade was 77.3% (187 of 241 patients) in our cohort (table 4). The most frequently reported drug-related AEs in patients treated with sorafenib were hand-foot skin reaction (109, 45.0%), diarrhea (76, 31.4%), hypertension (61, 25.2%), abnormal liver function (32, 13.2%), anorexia

Table 2. Univariate analysis of factors affecting OS

Factor/category	n	OS	95% CI	p value
Gender				
Male	180	16	9.6–18.6	
Female	61	10.3	7–21.2	0.9902
Age, years				
>73	119	15.6	10.1–21.7	
≤73	122	12.7	8.3–18.6	0.4632
Initial dose of sorafenib, mg				
≥400	114	16.1	10.3–21.6	
800	127	10.6	7.2–18.6	0.3683
Treatment duration, days				
>90	130	5.4	3.5–9.9	
≤90	111	21.7	18.6–26.8	<0.0001
Virus status				
Hepatitis B virus	43	18.3	6.4–28.3	
Hepatitis C virus	121	16.1	9.1–21.6	
Virus negative	77	9.2	6.9–18.6	0.1244
Up-to-7 criteria				
Within	64	26.9	19.9	
Out	177	8.3	6.4–11.8	<0.0001
Portal invasion				
No	173	18.3	12.7–21.3	
Yes	68	5.4	3.6–9.2	<0.0001
Extrahepatic spread				
No	169	16.7	11.3–21.6	
Yes	72	8.1	3.7–16	0.0018
PS				
0	225	16	10.3–19.4	
1	16	3.2	1.7–11.2	0.0113
Albumin, g/dl				
>3.5	109	8.1	5.9–11.3	
≤3.5	132	20.8	15.6–25.3	0.0004
Total bilirubin, mg/dl				
>1.0	148	18.8	15.6–24.7	
≤1.0	93	6	3.7–9.3	<0.0001
White blood cell count, /μl				
>5,000	123	18.6	15.6–24.2	
≤5,000	118	8.1	5.4–13.6	0.0172
Hemoglobin, g/dl				
>12	98	11.4	7.9–18.6	
≤12	143	16	8.8–21.2	0.4854
Platelet count, $\times 10^4$				
>15	136	17.4	11.3–22.8	
≤15	105	9.1	6.5–17.9	0.0335
ALT, IU/l				
>50	169	18.3	12.7–21.3	
≤50	72	8.1	5.8–11.3	0.0136
ALP, IU/l				
>400	116	18.3	13.6–21.6	
≤400	124	8.3	5.4–17.9	0.0163
AFP, ng/dl				
>400	139	19.4	16.1–24.7	
≤400	101	6.2	4.4–8.1	<0.0001
DCP, mAU/dl				
>1,000	111	21.3	17.4–25.4	
≤1,000	123	6.5	5.2–9.3	<0.0001
Alpha-fetoprotein L3, %				
>10	95	20.7	16.7–25.1	
≤10	136	9.2	6.9–16	0.0131
BCLC				
A or B	95	20.8	15.6–25.3	
C	146	9.2	6.5–13.6	0.0006
Child-Pugh score increase				
No	106	22.8	18.6–26.8	
+1≤ point	106	7.2	5.9–9.6	<0.0001
RECICL				
CR, PR, SD	135	20.7	16.7–26.9	
PD	86	7.3	6.0–1.8	<0.0001

Table 3. Multivariate analysis of factors affecting OS

Factor/category	p value	Hazard ratio	95% CI	
			lower limit	upper limit
Treatment duration, days				
>90	0.0204	1	0.3455	0.9143
≤90		0.5622		
Up-to-7 criteria				
Within	0.0400	1	1.0284	3.4947
Out		1.8655		
Child-Pugh score increase				
No	0.0008	1	1.3791	3.3955
+1≤ point		2.1575		
RECICL				
CR, PR, SD	0.0007	1	1.4077	3.5802
PD		2.2390		

(31, 12.8%), alopecia (11, 4.5%) and hoarseness (10, 4.1%). AEs of Grade 3 or more as defined by CTCAE v4.0 were observed in 23.6% (57 patients) of patients in our cohort: hand-foot skin reaction (28, 11.6%), liver dysfunction (12, 5.0%), hypertension (9, 3.7%), diarrhea (4, 1.7%), erythema multiforme (4, 1.7%), decreased platelet count (3, 1.2%), anorexia (2, 0.8%) and anemia (1, 0.4%).

Discussion

Since the demonstration of the efficacy of the molecular targeted agent sorafenib in the SHARP and the Asia-Pacific trials, various studies have reported on the efficacy of this drug. It has been 6 years since the approval of sorafenib in Japan. In the current study, we comprehen-

Table 4. Incidence of drug-related AEs

AE	Any grade	%	Grade 3 or more	%
Overall incidence	187	77.3	57	23.6
Hand-foot syndrome	109	45.0	28	11.6
Diarrhea	76	31.4	4	1.7
Hypertension	61	25.2	9	3.7
Liver dysfunction	32	13.2	12	5.0
Anorexia	31	12.8	2	0.8
Alopecia	11	4.5	0	0.0
Hoarseness	10	4.1	0	0.0
Decreased platelet count	9	3.7	3	1.2
Stomatitis	8	3.3	0	0.0
Erythema multiforme	6	2.5	4	1.7
Constipation	5	2.1	0	0.0
Nausea	4	1.7	0	0.0
Anemia	3	1.2	1	0.4
Interstitial pneumonia	2	0.8	0	0.0

sively analyzed the clinical course of all patients treated with sorafenib at our hospital and reported the treatment outcomes as well as the factors contributing to OS as a single-center experience.

The OS following sorafenib treatment was 14.3 months at our hospital, which was longer than that reported in the SHARP and the Asia-Pacific trials. The sorafenib-induced AEs of any grade were 77.3%, and Grade 3 or higher events accounted for 23.6%, demonstrating that AE outcomes were not greatly different from those of the SHARP and the Asia-Pacific trials [24, 25]. Furthermore, no remarkable difference was observed in comparison to the sorafenib-induced AEs reported in the GIDEON [27]. Our outcomes regarding AEs did not show great differences in comparison to other reports [38, 39], but the survival outcome in our study was superior to that of the SHARP and the Asia-Pacific trials [24, 25].

Currently, sorafenib is recommended for cases unresponsive to TACE [29]. TACE is considered to be effective for local control of the tumor. However, the multiple procedure of TACE should lead to deterioration of liver function where treatment with sorafenib could not be applicable; such a condition would result in the decrease of OS in HCC patients. Therefore, if the patient showed a poor tumor response to TACE, sorafenib treatment is strongly recommended instead of continuing TACE even if the patient is still in an early stage. The relatively early induction of sorafenib for patients who did not respond to TACE could be a cause of longer survival in our study as compared to other studies.

The results of this study showed that factors contributing to survival include the administration period of sorafenib, up-to-7 criteria, change in Child-Pugh score and response evaluation. Sorafenib could induce several antitumor effects, including tumor necrosis; the increase of OS, which is the most important outcome of sorafenib treatment, should be attributed to the inhibition of tumor proliferation [40]. Therefore, long-term administration with control AE should be critical to extract the potential of sorafenib even in cases with SD. Furthermore, as the decrease in the Child-Pugh score results in the decrease in OS, the preservation of liver function is also important in addition to the control of AEs. As there is a report claiming that branched chain amino acid preparations are effective in preventing decreases in the albumin levels during sorafenib administration [41], it is also necessary to take a supportive therapy to preserve liver function.

Based on our experience with a large number of cases, we conclude that contentious treatment with sorafenib for a long period is critical to extract the maximum efficacy even if SD or a more favorable outcome is obtained, because sorafenib is the only molecular targeted drug that has demonstrated efficacy for advanced HCC, and there is no second-line therapy with sorafenib.

Disclosure Statement

Authors declare no conflict of interest.

References

1 Llovet JM, Burroughs A, Bruix J: Hepatocellular carcinoma. Lancet 2003;362:1907–1917.
2 Belghiti J, Fuks D: Liver resection and transplantation in hepatocellular carcinoma. Liver Cancer 2012;1:71–82.
3 Shindoh J, Kaseb A, Vauthey JN: Surgical strategy for liver cancers in the era of effective chemotherapy. Liver Cancer 2013;2:47–54.
4 Mise Y, Sakamoto Y, Ishizawa T, et al: A worldwide survey of the current daily practice in liver surgery. Liver Cancer 2013;2:55–66.
5 Lee Cheah Y, K H Chow P: Liver transplantation for hepatocellular carcinoma: an appraisal of current controversies. Liver Cancer 2012;1:183–189.
6 Chan SC: Liver transplantation for hepatocellular carcinoma. Liver Cancer 2013;2:338–344.
7 Chan SC, Sharr WW, Chan AC, et al: Rescue living-donor liver transplantation for liver failure following hepatectomy for hepatocellular carcinoma. Liver Cancer 2013;2:332–337.
8 Akamatsu N, Sugawara Y, Kokudo N: Living donor liver transplantation for patients with hepatocellular carcinoma. Liver Cancer 2014;3:108–118.

9 Bruix J, Llovet JM: Prognostic prediction and treatment strategy in hepatocellular carcinoma. Hepatology 2002;35:519–524.
10 Park KW, Park JW, Choi JI, et al: Survival analysis of 904 patients with hepatocellular carcinoma in a hepatitis B virus-endemic area. J Gastroenterol Hepatol 2008;23:467–473.
11 Lin SM: Local ablation for hepatocellular carcinoma in Taiwan. Liver Cancer 2013;2:73–83.
12 Teng W, Liu KW, Lin CC, et al: Insufficient ablative margin determined by early computed tomography may predict the recurrence of hepatocellular carcinoma after radiofrequency ablation. Liver Cancer 2015;4:26–38.
13 Kudo M: Locoregional therapy for hepatocellular carcinoma. Liver Cancer 2015;4:163–164.
14 Lencioni R: Chemoembolization in patients with hepatocellular carcinoma. Liver Cancer 2012;1:41–50.
15 Raoul JL, Gilabert M, Piana G: How to define transarterial chemoembolization failure or refractoriness: a European perspective. Liver Cancer 2014;3:119–124.
16 Minami Y, Yagyu Y, Murakami T, et al: Tracking navigation imaging of transcatheter arterial chemoembolization for hepatocellular carcinoma using three-dimensional cone-beam CT angiography. Liver Cancer 2014;3:53–61.
17 Kudo M: Treatment of advanced hepatocellular carcinoma with emphasis on hepatic arterial infusion chemotherapy and molecular targeted therapy. Liver Cancer 2012;1:62–70.
18 Lin S, Hoffmann K, Schemmer P: Treatment of hepatocellular carcinoma: a systematic review. Liver Cancer 2012;1:144–158.
19 Peck-Radosavljevic M: Drug therapy for advanced-stage liver cancer. Liver Cancer 2014;3:125–131.
20 Benson AB 3rd, Abrams TA, Ben-Josef E, et al: NCCN clinical practice guidelines in oncology: hepatobiliary cancers. J Natl Compr Canc Netw 2009;7:350–391.
21 European Association for the Study of the Liver; European Organisation for Research and Treatment of Cancer: EASL-EORTC clinical practice guidelines: management of hepatocellular carcinoma. J Hepatol 2012;56:908–943.
22 Verslype C, Rosmorduc O, Rougier P; ESMO Guidelines Working Group: Hepatocellular carcinoma: ESMO-ESDO clinical practice guidelines for diagnosis, treatment and follow-up. Ann Oncol 2012;23(suppl 7):vii41–vii48.
23 Kudo M, Matsui O, Izumi N, et al: Transarterial chemoembolization failure/refractoriness: JSH-LCSGJ criteria 2014 update. Oncology 2014;87(suppl 1):22–31.
24 Llovet JM, Ricci S, Mazzaferro V, et al: Sorafenib in advanced hepatocellular carcinoma. N Engl J Med 2008;359:378–390.
25 Cheng AL, Kang YK, Chen Z, et al: Efficacy and safety of sorafenib in patients in the Asia-Pacific region with advanced hepatocellular carcinoma: a phase III randomised, double-blind, placebo-controlled trial. Lancet Oncol 2009;10:25–34.
26 Lencioni R, Kudo M, Ye SL, et al: First interim analysis of the GIDEON (global investigation of therapeutic decisions in hepatocellular carcinoma and of its treatment with sorafenib) non-interventional study. Int J Clin Pract 2012;66:675–683.
27 Lencioni R, Kudo M, Ye SL, et al: GIDEON (global investigation of therapeutic decisions in hepatocellular carcinoma and of its treatment with sorafenib): second interim analysis. Int J Clin Pract 2014;68:609–617.
28 Kudo M, Izumi N, Kokudo N, et al: Management of hepatocellular carcinoma in Japan: consensus-based clinical practice guidelines proposed by the Japan society of hepatology (JSH) 2010 updated version. Dig Dis 2011;29:339–364.
29 Arizumi T, Ueshima K, Chishina H, et al: Validation of the criteria of transcatheter arterial chemoembolization failure or refractoriness in patients with advanced hepatocellular carcinoma proposed by the LCSGJ. Oncology 2014;87(suppl 1):32–36.
30 Ogasawara S, Chiba T, Ooka Y, et al: Efficacy of sorafenib in intermediate-stage hepatocellular carcinoma patients refractory to transarterial chemoembolization. Oncology 2014;87:330–341.
31 Kudo M, Ueshima K, Arizumi T: Real-life clinical practice with sorafenib in advanced hepatocellular carcinoma: a single-center experience. Dig Dis 2012;30:609–616.
32 Kudo M: Alpha-fetoprotein-L3: useful or useless for hepatocellular carcinoma? Liver Cancer 2013;2:151–152.
33 Song P, Gao J, Inagaki Y, et al: Biomarkers: evaluation of screening for and early diagnosis of hepatocellular carcinoma in Japan and China. Liver Cancer 2013;2:31–39.
34 Toyoda H, Kumada T, Tada T, et al: Tumor markers for hepatocellular carcinoma: simple and significant predictors of outcome in patients with HCC. Liver Cancer 2015;4:126–136.
35 Llovet JM, Brú C, Bruix J: Prognosis of hepatocellular carcinoma: the BCLC staging classification. Semin Liver Dis 1999;19:329–338.
36 Kudo M, Ueshima K, Kubo S, et al: Response evaluation criteria in cancer of the liver (RECICL) (2015 revised version). Hepatol Res 2015, Epub ahead of print.
37 Mazzaferro V, Llovet JM, Miceli R, et al: Predicting survival after liver transplantation in patients with hepatocellular carcinoma beyond the Milan criteria: a retrospective, exploratory analysis. Lancet Oncol 2009;10:35–43.
38 Nishikawa H, Takeda H, Tsuchiya K, et al: Sorafenib therapy for BCLC stage B/C hepatocellular carcinoma; clinical outcome and safety in aged patients: a multicenter study in Japan. J Cancer 2014;5:499–509.
39 Jo M, Yasui K, Kirishima T, et al: Efficacy and safety of sorafenib in very elderly patients aged 80 years and older with advanced hepatocellular carcinoma. Hepatol Res 2014;44:1329–1338.
40 Arizumi T, Ueshima K, Chishina H, et al: Duration of stable disease is associated with overall survival in patients with advanced hepatocellular carcinoma treated with sorafenib. Dig Dis 2014;32:705–710.
41 Takeda H, Nishikawa H, Iguchi E, et al: Effect of treatment with branched-chain amino acids during sorafenib therapy for unresectable hepatocellular carcinoma. Hepatol Res 2014;44:302–312.

Original Article

Digestive Diseases

Dig Dis 2015;33:735–744
DOI: 10.1159/000439097

Cholangiocarcinoma in Cirrhosis: Value of Hepatocyte Specific Magnetic Resonance Imaging

Fabio Piscaglia[a] Massimo Iavarone[b] Marzia Galassi[a] Sara Vavassori[b] Matteo Renzulli[c] Laura Virginia Forzenigo[d] Alessandro Granito[a] Veronica Salvatore[a] Angelo Sangiovanni[b] Rita Golfieri[c] Massimo Colombo[b] Luigi Bolondi[a]

[a]Division of Internal Medicine, University of Bologna, S. Orsola-Malpighi Hospital, Bologna, [b]A.M. and A. Migliavacca Center for Liver Disease, 1st Division of Gastroenterology, Fondazione IRCCS Ca' Granda Maggiore Hospital, University of Milan, Milan, [c]Radiology Unit, General and University S. Orsola-Malpighi Hospital, Bologna, and [d]Division of Radiology, Fondazione IRCCS Ca' Granda Maggiore Hospital, Milan, Italy

Key Words
Cirrhosis · Contrast media · Differential diagnosis · Hepatocellular carcinoma · Liver cancer

Abstract
Background: The diagnosis of intrahepatic cholangiocellular carcinoma (ICC) remains elusive at imaging, which is a critical issue in cirrhotic patients in whom a diagnosis of hepatocellular carcinoma (HCC) can be established only by imaging. ***Aim:*** The aim of the study was to evaluate the potential of MRI in the diagnosis of ICC in cirrhosis using 'hepatocyte-specific' Gadolinium (Gd)-based contrast agents. ***Methods:*** Sixteen histologically proven and retrospectively identified ICCs on cirrhosis were investigated with hepatocyte-specific magnetic resonance contrast agents (6 in Bologna with Gd-EOB-DTPA and 10 in Milan with Gd-BOPTA). The control group consisted of 41 consecutively and prospectively collected nodules (31 HCCs) imaged with Gd-EOB-DTPA. ***Results:*** Fifteen ICC nodules (94%) displayed hypointensity in the hepatobiliary phase, suggesting malignancy. Thirteen cholangiocarcinomas (81%) showed hyperenhancement in the venous phase. Only 2 cholangiocarcinoma nodules showed hypoenhancement in the venous phase, corresponding to washout, in both cases preceded by rim enhancement in arterial phase. All the hepatocarcinomas showed hypointensity in hepatobiliary phase, but was always preceded by hypointensity in the venous phase; arterial rim enhancement was never observed in any hepatocarcinoma or regenerative nodule. ***Conclusions:*** MRI with hepatocyte-specific Gd-based contrast agents showed a pattern of malignancy in almost all the ICCs, concurrently avoiding misdiagnosis with hepatocarcinoma. These findings suggest a greater diagnostic capacity for this technique compared with the results of MRI with conventional contrast agents reported in the literature in this setting. © 2015 S. Karger AG, Basel

Introduction

The diagnosis of small hepatocellular carcinoma (HCC) in cirrhosis may be achieved by contrast imaging alone [1], yet it is challenged by the occurrence of non-

KARGER 125

© 2015 S. Karger AG, Basel
0257–2753/15/0336–0735$39.50/0

E-Mail karger@karger.com
www.karger.com/ddi

Prof. Fabio Piscaglia
Division Internal Medicine
Via Albertoni 15
IT–40138 Bologna (Italy)
E-Mail fabio.piscaglia@unibo.it

neoplastic nodules and peripheral intrahepatic cholangiocellular carcinoma (ICC) [2, 3], the latter occurring at a rate of 1–2% of new nodules in cirrhosis [4–7]. Indeed, MRI is the imaging technique of choice to suggest ICC in cirrhosis by showing peripheral enhancement of the nodule during the arterial phase coupled with the absence of a global washout in the venous phase [2], a finding however that increases the risk of misdiagnosis with such benign lesions, as hypervascular hemangioma and wash-in positive dysplastic hepatocellular macronodules [8, 9] and that requires liver biopsy, whenever feasible, to obtain a conclusive diagnosis.

MRI with hepatocyte-specific contrast agents, including Gadoxetic acid (Gd-EOB-DTPA, Primovist®, Bayer-Shering, Germany) or Gadobenate dimeglumine (Gd-BOPTA, Multihance®, Bracco, Milan, Italy) is gaining popularity in increasing the sensitivity of non-invasive approaches to diagnose HCC. These contrast agents serve the purpose of depicting both the vascular and the hepatobiliary phases of MRI [10–13], and they provide the same type of information, although the acquisition timing schedules of the 2 are different according to the different pharmacokinetics. The contrast medium is taken up by physiologically functioning hepatocytes, whereas malignant nodules present enhancement defects during the hepatobiliary phase of enhancement due to the lack of such function in tumoral cells [14–19]. The Japanese Society of Hepatology had already endorsed the use of hepatocyte-specific MRI contrast agents for the diagnosis of HCC in patients with cirrhosis in the previous set of recommendations [20] and has extended it in the most recent update [21]. However, the issue of the patterns displayed by other primary liver malignancies that may arise in cirrhosis [22] and their appearance at hepatocyte-specific contrast MRI is not mentioned in these guidelines. Indeed, the potential of hepatocyte-specific MRI contrast agents to diagnose ICC has never been investigated specifically in the setting of patients with cirrhosis. This population is peculiar as hepatocellular uptake and biliary excretion of the contrast agents might be impaired [15], and the fibrous rich stroma of ICC might bind gadolinium [23] and prolong enhancement to an unknown extent. Thus, although it has already been reported that ICC in general tend to show enhancement defect in the hepatobiliary phase of contrast imaging, such findings have not yet been specifically reported in patients with cirrhosis, despite contrast imaging of focal liver lesions follows distinct flow charts for patients with or without cirrhosis [24]. Indeed, data valid in patients with normal liver cannot be straightforwardly assumed also for cirrhotic patients. For instance, a recent article on contrast-enhanced ultrasound patterns of ICC showed different prevalence of contrast patterns in patients with or without a background of cirrhosis [25].

The aim of the present study was to evaluate whether ICC can be reliably diagnosed using MRI with hepatocyte-specific contrast agents in patients with cirrhosis.

Patients and Methods

Patients

A retrospective search utilizing pathology files, clinical unit databases and needle biopsy reports was conducted for cirrhotic patients diagnosed with ICC at S. Orsola-Malpighi Hospital in Bologna during 2008–2013 (when the hepatobiliary MRI contrast agent Gd-EOB-DTPA became available). Patients with ICC on cirrhosis were identified in Milan by retrospective scrutiny of fine needle biopsy reports in patients presenting at the Liver Center at Fondazione IRCCS Ca' Granda Maggiore Hospital. The study protocol was approved by the institutional review boards. Informed consent was requested only for patients who were still alive given the retrospective nature of the studies. The stage of the underlying liver disease as cirrhotic or severe fibrotic (categories at risk for HCC according to international guidelines) [21, 26, 27] was established by biopsy or by consistent clinical, laboratory, ultrasonographic and/or endoscopic findings, according to accepted guidelines [28].

A total of 15 cirrhotic patients with ICC were identified in Bologna of which 6 (1 nodule each) had been investigated by MRI also with Gd-EOB-DTPA for diagnostic and staging purposes (subgroup A). A total of 19 patients with ICC were identified in Milan and 7 (with a total of 10 ICC nodules) investigated by Gd-BOPTA MRI (subgroup B). The MRI patterns of all the 16 ICC nodules were reviewed. Eleven of 13 patients had early stage tumors, as per the Barcelona Clinic Liver Cancer staging system for HCC [26] (table 1). In subgroup A, 4 patients were under surveillance for HCC, whereas 2 patients had incidental histological diagnosis of ICC and cirrhosis during surgical resection.

All 7 patients in subgroup B were under regular surveillance for cirrhosis. At the time of diagnosis, 1 patient had 3 simultaneous nodules localized in different segments of the liver that were each histologically characterized by fine needle biopsy as ICC (patient subgroup B-11). These 3 nodules were assessed separately. In another patient, under surveillance following hepatic resection of an ICC, a second nodule of ICC was histologically diagnosed 4 years later (patient subgroup B-13). The imaging patterns of these 2 liver nodules were assessed separately.

Five patients from subgroup A and 4 from subgroup B underwent surgical resection, with ICC confirmed at pathology. The remaining patients in subgroup A received endoarterial radioembolization with Yttrium 90 after bioptic diagnosis of ICC, whereas the non-surgical patients in subgroup B were treated by radiofrequency ablation (2 de novo detected + 1 recurrence) or chemotherapy (n = 1).

The enhancement patterns of the ICC group were compared with those of the control group consisting of patients, included in a prospective study run in Bologna on the use of imaging techniques in 41 small nodules (10–30 mm), selected because they con-

Table 1. Demography and tumor characteristics of patients with ICC

Patient	Age	Sex	Etiology of liver disease	Child-Pugh class	Lesion number	ICC size, mm	Liver segment	Surveillance	Segmental bile duct dilation
Subgroup A-1	70	Male	Alcohol	A	1	30	3	No	No
Subgroup A-2	70	Male	Crypto	A	1	32	5	Yes	Yes
Subgroup A-3	52	Male	Alcohol	A	1	35	4	Yes	No
Subgroup A-4	65	Male	HBV	A	1	50	7–8	Yes	Yes
Subgroup A-5	66	Male	HCV	A	1 ICC 1 HCC	21 18	4 2	No	No
Subgroup A-6	60	Female	HBV	A	1	50	6–7	No	No
Subgroup B-7	63	Male	HCV	A	1	23	2	Yes	No
Subgroup B-8	59	Male	HCV + alcohol	A	1	16	8	Yes	No
Subgroup B-9	60	Male	HCV + alcohol	A	1	24	8	Yes	No
Subgroup B-10	70	Male	HCV	A	1	20	4	Yes	No
Subgroup B-11	77	Female	Alcohol	A	1 2 3	85 15 20	6 4 2	Yes	Yes
Subgroup B-12	62	Male	HCV	A	1	58	8	Yes	No
Subgroup B-13	69	Male	HBV	A	1	30	5	Yes	No
Subgroup B-13	73	Male	HBV	A	1	30	7	Yes	No

Subgroup A = Patients enrolled in Bologna; Subgroup B = patients enrolled in Milan; HBV = hepatitis B virus; HCV = hepatitis C virus.

secutively submitted to MRI with the hepato-specific contrast agent Gd-EOB-DTPA [29]. The nodules were initially detected during ultrasonographic surveillance in 26 cirrhotic patients between 2008 and 2010. The histological diagnosis in this series was of 31 HCCs and 10 regenerative nodules either with or without dysplasia (3 non-malignant confirmed at histology, the remaining by a stable size over a follow-up of at least 24 months).

Informed consent was obtained by patients, whenever possible, according to the recommendation of the ethics committee in agreement with the retrospective study design.

Methods

In Bologna, MRI was carried out with a 1.5-tesla superconducting system (Signa, GE Medical Systems, Milwaukee, Wis., USA), using a body phased-array multicoil for signal detection, as previously described [19]. Images were acquired in the axial plane, with a section thickness of 4 mm, an intersection gap of 0 mm and a 28–35 cm field of view, with the exception of a 3-dimensional (3D) breath-hold fast spoiled gradient-echo (GRE) sequence obtained after Gd-EOB-DTPA injection, acquired with a slice thickness of 4–5 mm and an effective section thickness of 2–2.5 mm. Contrast-enhanced sequences were acquired after an intravenous injection of Gd-EOB-DTPA at a dose of 0.1 ml/kg body weight (injection volume of 9–14 ml according to body weight) at a speed of 1–2 ml/s immediately followed by a 20 ml saline flush through an antecubital venous catheter, using a dual power injector. Both dynamic and hepatobiliary phase images were obtained using a fat-suppressed 3D GRE sequence (Liver Acquisition with Volume Acceleration: LAVA, GE Medical Systems) before and after intravenous bolus administration of Gd-EOB-DTPA. Imaging delay times were determined with real-time MRI fluoroscopic monitoring after the administration of contrast agent. Hepatic arterial phase images were obtained 7 s after the contrast medium had reached the distal thoracic aorta, and portal venous and equilibrium phase images were obtained 60 and 180 s, respectively, after the beginning of the injection. Finally, hepatobiliary phase imaging was obtained 10 and 20 min after the beginning of contrast medium injection. Images reviews were performed by an experienced radiologist (M.R.), in keeping with the AASLD guidelines [30]. In Milan, MRI was carried out with a 1.5-tesla system (Avanto, Siemens Medical Systems, Erlangen, Germany) using a phased-array torso coil for signal detection, as previously described [6]. All the patients underwent transverse T1- and T2-weighted MRI and multiphasic contrast-enhanced dynamic 3D MRI of the whole liver with fat suppression. T1-weighted imaging included breath-hold in-phase GRE (175/5 TR/TE, 256 × 112 matrix, 70° flip angle) and out-of-phase GRE (175/2.38 TR/TE, 256 × 112 matrix, 70° flip angle). T2-weighted imaging included fat suppression sequences (1310/70 TR/TE, 320 × 192 matrix). Dynamic MRI was carried out with a 3D Volumetric Interpolated Breath-hold Examination (VIBE) sequence in the axial plane by using the following parameters: 4.7/2.3, 10° flip angle, 320 × 157 matrix, slice thickness of 3 mm. Gd-BOPTA was injected at a dose of 0.2 ml/kg at a rate of 2 ml/s. Arterial, portal venous and late venous phase images were ac-

Table 2. MRI findings in ICC nodules after intravenous contrast enhancement in arterial, portal and post-vascular hepato-specific phases

Patient	Weighted T1 image	Weighted T2 image	Arterial phase	Portal phase	Late venous phase	Hepatobiliary post-vascular phase
Subgroup A-1	Hypointense	Hyperintense	Hyperenhancement	Hyperenhancement	Slight Non-homogeneous Hyperenhancement	Enhancement defect
Subgroup A-2	Slightly hypointense	Hypointense	Rim enhancement	Centripetal enhancement	Hyperenhancement	Enhancement defect
Subgroup A-3	Hypointense	Hyperintense	Rim enhancement	Centripetal enhancement	Hyperenhancement	Enhancement defect
Subgroup A-4	Hypointense	Hyperintense	Rim enhancement	Centripetal enhancement	Hyperenhancement	Enhancement defect
Subgroup A-5	Hypointense	Hyperintense	Slightly hyperenhancement	Hyperenhancement	Hyperenhancement	Enhancement defect
Subgroup A-6	Hypointense	Hyperintense	Non-homogeneous hyperenhancement	Centripetal enhancement	Hyperenhancement	Enhancement defect
Subgroup B-7	Slightly hypointense	Hyperintense	Rim enhancement	Hypoenhancement	Hypoenhancement	Enhancement defect
Subgroup B-8	Hypointense	Hyperintense	Hyperenhancement	Hyperenhancement	Hyperenhancement	Enhancement defect
Subgroup B-9	Hyperintense	Isointense	Isoenhancement	Isoenhancement	Isoenhancement	Enhancement defect
Subgroup B-10	Hypointense	Hyperintense	Rim enhancement	Rim enhancement	Rim enhancement	Enhancement defect (Rim)
Subgroup B-11	Hypointense	Hyperintense	Non-homogeneous hyperenhancement	Non-homogeneous hyperenhancement	Non-homogeneous hyperenhancement	Enhancement defect
	Hypointense	Hyperintense	Hyperenhancement	Hyperenhancement	Hyperenhancement	Enhancement defect
	Hypointense	Hyperintense	Hyperenhancement	Hyperenhancement	Hyperenhancement	Enhancement defect
Subgroup B-12	Hypointense	Hyperintense	Hypoenhancement	Hypoenhancement	Hyperenhancement	Enhancement defect
Subgroup B-13	Hyperintense	Hyperintense	Non-homogenous hyperenhancement	Non-homogenous hyperenhancement	Hyperenhancement	Isoenhancement
Subgroup B-13	Hypointense	Hyperintense	Rim enhancement	Hypoenhancement	Hypoenhancement	Enhancement defect

quired approximately 30, 80 and 180 s from the start of the contrast injection, respectively. A breath-hold T1-weighted 2D GRE with fat suppression MRI (4.7/2.3 TR/TE, 256 × 157 matrix) and 3D VIBE sequences were carried out 2 h after contrast injection (hepatobiliary phase).

The timing schedules utilized with the 2 MRI contrast agents were different to reflect the different pharmacokinetics, but each was in keeping with the regular standard practice for that agent, so that the acquisitions were expected to produce exactly the same type of results, allowing the combining of findings obtained with the 2 agents. Images reviews were performed by an experienced radiologist (L.V.F.) who was blinded to biopsy results.

Results are reported in an extensive descriptive modality.

Results

A majority of ICC patients had alcohol-related (38.5%) cirrhosis (table 1), whereas alcohol etiology represented only a minority of the patients with hepatocellular lesions, either HCC or regenerative nodules, seen in Bologna. Thus, alcohol-related cirrhosis was significantly more associated to ICC than to hepatocellular lesions, (38.5 vs. 3.9%, $p < 0.05$). All other patient characteristics were not statistically different.

The results of imaging techniques in ICC nodules (median size 30 mm) are reported in table 2. During the vascular phases of the study, a total of 6 nodules (38%) showed rim enhancement, 8 (50%) hyperenhancement (5 homogenous and 3 non-homogenous), 1 (6%) was isoenhancing and 1 (6%) was hypoenhancing in the arterial phase. In the venous phase, 13 nodules (81%) showed hyperenhancement (12 homogeneous and 1 with only rim-like enhancement; fig. 1 and 2). Only 2 ICC nodules showed washout in the venous phase, which was preceded by rim-like enhancement in the arterial phase (table 2; fig. 1), therefore not associated with the typical HCC hallmark consisting of homogeneous hyperenhancement in

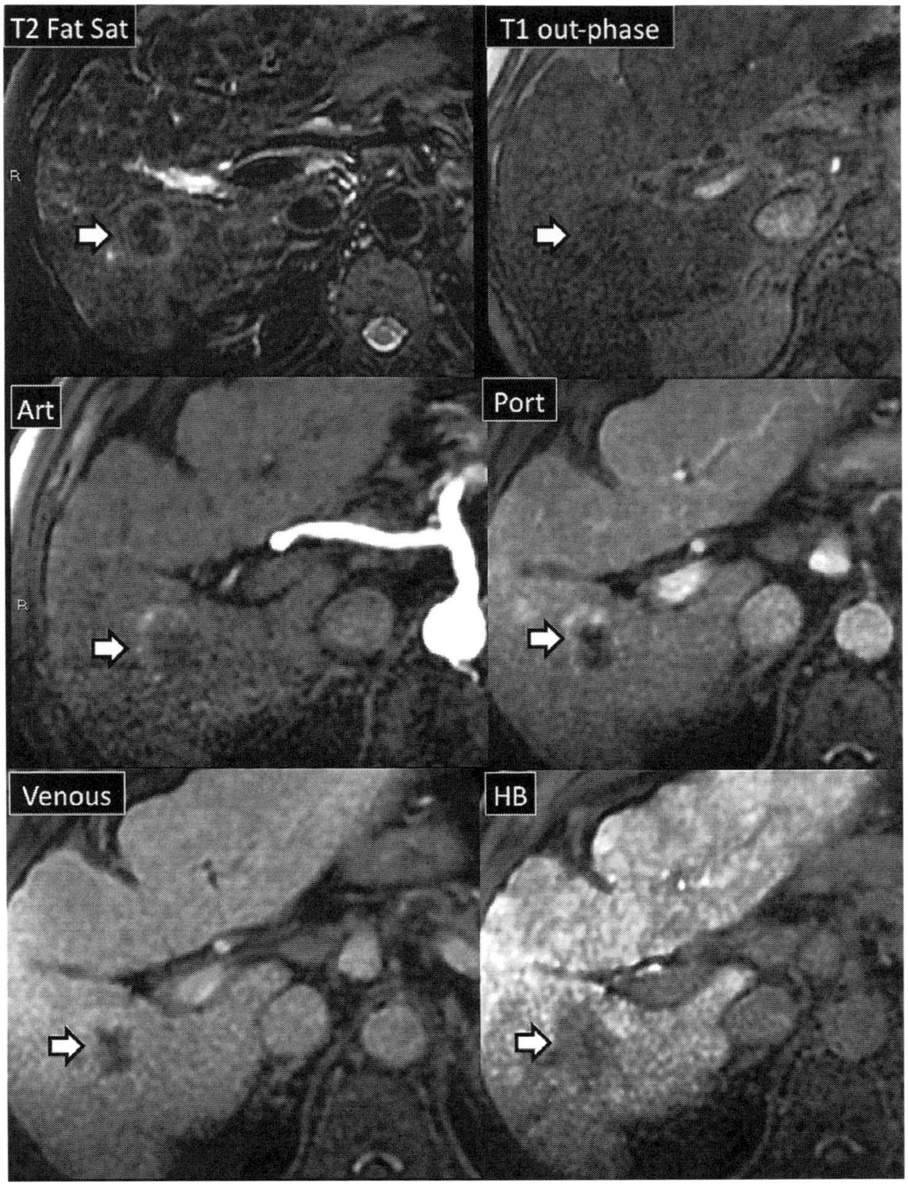

Fig. 1. ICC assessed by MRI with Gd-EOB-DTPA (Primovist) showing T2 hyperintensity during the pre-contrast phase T2 (FatSat FRFSE T2-weighted), whereas the pattern is slightly hypo in out-of-phase T1. A peripheral hyperenhancement seen in the arterial phase persists in the portal and late venous phases, without any washout, whereas the center of the lesion is continuously hypointense. In the hepatobiliary phase (HB), the nodule becomes an enhancement defect comprising both the peripheral and the central portions.

the arterial phase followed by homogeneous washout in the venous phase. The remaining nodule was isoenhancing in all the vascular phases.

All but 1 (94%) ICC nodule showed an enhancement defect during the hepatobiliary phase (fig. 1, 2).

The analysis of the dynamic enhancement pattern throughout the vascular and hepatobiliary phases of the study in 14 of 16 (88%) ICC nodules showed a sequence of features not observed in any hepatocellular nodule, whether malignant or not. The 2 additional nodules were as follows: one showed a progressive increase in enhancement from the arterial to the venous phase, followed by isoenhancement in the hepatobiliary phase, and the other one showed isoenhancement throughout all the vascular phases, followed by an enhancement defect in the hepatobiliary phase. Thus, the former did not show any feature of malignancy at all, and the latter showed a pattern that is observed also in dysplastic regenerative nodules or in early HCC (table 3).

Indeed, in the control group, an enhancement defect in the hepatobiliary phase was found in all 31 (100%) of the HCC nodules and in 3 (30%) of the non-malignant nodules (table 3). Importantly, the enhancement defect

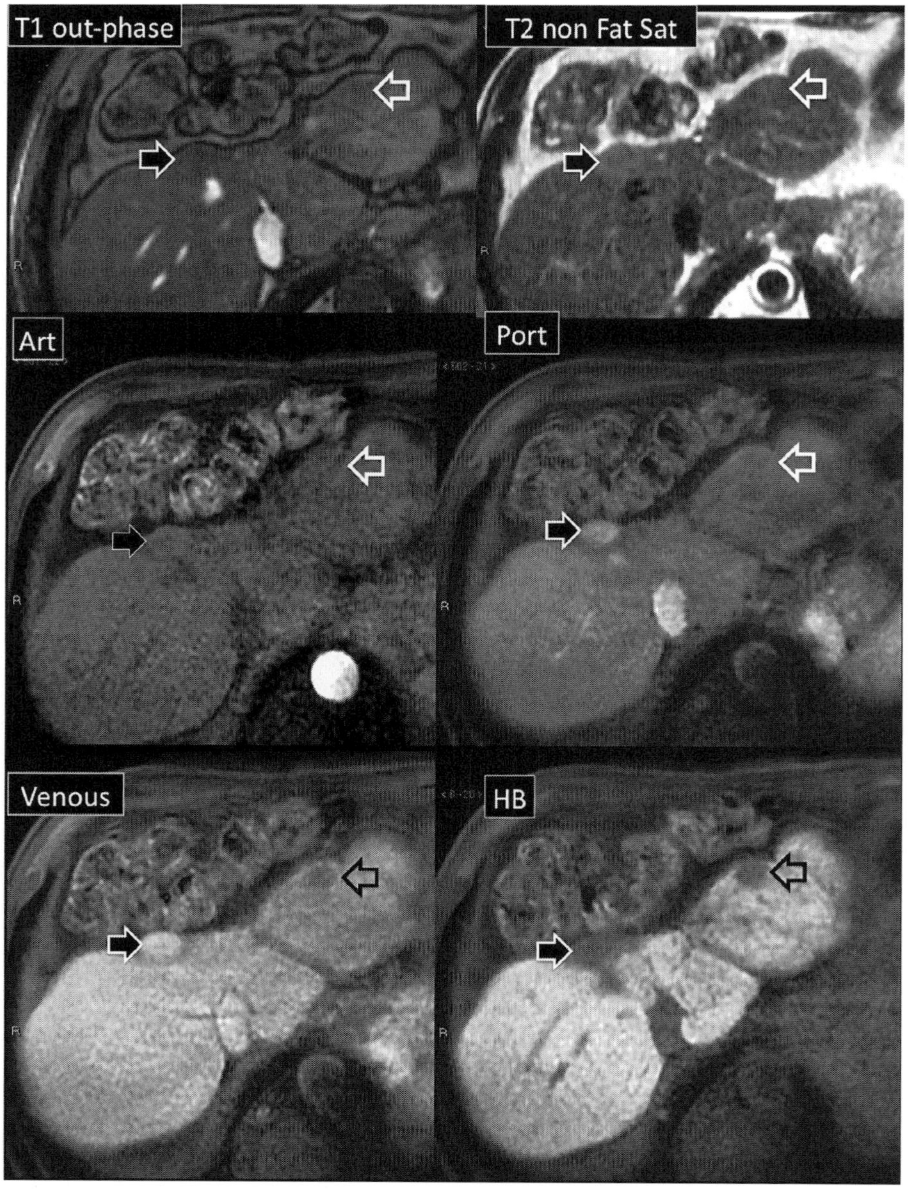

Fig. 2. The patient depicted in this figure concurrently had an ICC (full black arrows) in segment 4 and an HCC in segment 2 (empty arrows), each showing a distinct contrast pattern. The images were taken during MRI with Gd-EOB-DTPA (Primovist). The T2 pre-contrast images were acquired with a non-FatSat SSFSE sequence. In the arterial phase, the ICC appears isoenhancing, whereas a progressive increase in enhancement occurs in the portal and late phases leading to hyperenhancement (best visible in the portal phase). No washout appeared. Conversely, the HCC nodule is isoenhancing in the arterial phase, likewise ICC, but it shows hypoenhancement in the venous phase. Both tumor nodules appear as enhancement defects in the hepatobiliary phase (HB).

was preceded by washout in the venous vascular phase in all HCC nodules (100%), but only in 2 of 15 (13%) ICC nodules with a post-vascular enhancement defect (tables 2 and 3). Moreover, as previously mentioned, these 2 ICC nodules showing venous washout followed by hepatobiliary enhancement defect had a rim-like hyperenhancement during the arterial phase, a pattern never observed in any HCC or regenerative nodule. Thus, almost no overlap was observed between the appearance of cholangiocellular and hepatocellular focal lesions at MRI with hepatobiliary contrast agents, apart from the few ones with a persistent isoenhancement in all vascular phases followed by hepatobiliary enhancement defect, which would anyhow require biopsy, since lacking any arterial hyperenhancement (table 3).

Discussion

This study showed characteristic findings for ICC in cirrhosis using MRI with hepatocyte-specific Gadolinium (Gd)-based contrast agents. This consisted of rim-like or diffuse arterial hyperenhancement, followed by either a progressive increase in enhancement or a sustained en-

Table 3. Contrast imaging patterns defined according to the degree of enhancement in the vascular and post-vascular phases in different types of nodules in cirrhosis, explored by MRI with hepatobiliary phase contrast agents

Enhancement patterns			Type of lesion		
arterial	venous	hepatobiliary phase	ICC (n = 16)	HCC (n = 31)	non-malignant (n = 10)
↑ (Rim)	↑	↓ (E-defect)	4	0	0
↑ (Rim)	=	↓ (E-defect)	0	0	0
↑ (Rim)	↓	↓ (E-defect)	2	0	0
↑	↑	↓ (E-defect)	8	0	0
↑	=	↓ (E-defect)	0	0	0
↑	↓	↓ (E-defect)	0	24	0
=	↑	↓ (E-defect)	0	0	0
=	=	**↓ (E-defect)**	**1**	0	**3**
=	↓	↓ (E-defect)	0	7	0
= or ↓	=	=	0	0	10
↓	↑	↓ (E-defect)	1	0	0
↓	↓	↓ (E-defect)	0	0	0
↑ or ↓	↑ or ↓	=	0	0	0

hancement in the portal/late venous phases followed by an enhancement defect in the post-vascular hepatobiliary phase.

The current findings are in agreement with what could have been theoretically expected, but never have been previously demonstrated in the setting of the diagnostic strategy of nodules in cirrhosis, since the only previous study demonstrating the enhancement defect pattern in the post-vascular phase of ICC did not include patients with small nodules detected in cirrhosis, leaving unanswered the question addressed by the present work [31].

One major concern in the imaging of ICC by hepatocyte-specific contrast MRI in cirrhosis was the known possibility of Gd-based contrast agents to bind to fibrous tissue [32, 33], including the fibrous-rich matrix present in ICC [23] as well as the fibrotic liver itself. On one side, this behavior makes the diagnosis of HCC easier [19, 34], as it is poor in fibrous tissue and surrounded by fibrotic cirrhotic parenchyma, but on the other side, this property could theoretically make it difficult to distinguish ICC, given its fibrous matrix, from the surrounding fibrotic liver [15]. Our observation of an enhancement defect in the hepatobiliary phase in patients with sustained enhancement in the late vascular phase suggests that Gad binds to the fibrous matrix of ICC only transiently, hence not preventing the typical pattern of malignancy to be detected during the hepatobiliary post-vascular phase also in this type of cancer. This is not a trivial finding since the sustained enhancement in the late vascular phase in ICC indeed prevents a misdiagnosis of HCC [2], but in cases of biopsy unfeasibility, may expose the patient to the risk of a false diagnosis of non-malignant nodule, since washout in the late venous phase is considered a cornerstone for the diagnosis of malignancy [30, 35]. Thus, the identification of an additional contrast feature, reinforcing the suspicion of malignancy in patients lacking washout would be very important and warranted. The present study showed that the enhancement defect in the hepatobiliary phase could represent this additional feature in patients with ICC.

It is worth to remark that the findings expected in HCC [36, 37] and endorsed by the various editions of Japanese HCC guidelines (enhancement defect in the hepatobiliary phase) [20, 27, 38] could not be assumed to surely occur in ICC also, although both are malignant lesions with loss of hepatocyte function. In fact, ICC is different from HCC in that it is often associated with desmoplastic reaction [39] and Gd tends to bind to fibrous tissue [32, 33], hence making the possibility of not observing an enhancement defect in the post-vascular phase real. Thus, a demonstration of the post-vascular pattern of ICC in cirrhosis (where imaging diagnosis of tumors is accepted, differently from almost all other instances) was necessary.

The pattern of arterial hyperenhancement followed by sustained or increasing enhancement up to the late venous phase coupled with enhancement defect in the hepatobiliary phase can be found in hypervascular hemangioma [40]. However, the pre-contrast MRI pattern is usually highly diagnostic for hemangioma, thus avoiding a misdiagnosis with hepatocellular or biliary lesions [41–43]. Moreover, had any case remained not clarified about whether it is hemangioma or ICC, contrast-enhanced ultrasound can easily distinguish between the them [24]. Once hemangioma is excluded, the risk of malignancy is foreseen by the detection of enhancement defect in the hepatobiliary phase at MRI [14–19, 36] which, in fact, was present practically in all our HCCs or ICCs.

While HCC is diagnosed by the presence of washout in the portal/venous phases following hyperenhancement in the arterial phase [30] and by an enhancement defect in the post-vascular phase, Japanese experts also consider a 'corona' enhancement in the late arterial or portal venous phase as diagnostic for HCC [20]. However, 'corona' enhancement is typically characteristic for HCC where the appearance of washout in the late venous phase takes place [20], a pattern never observed in our ICC at

Dig Dis 2015;33:735–744
DOI: 10.1159/000439097

MRI, despite the possible presence of peripheral enhancement in the arterial or portal phases (fig. 1). The MRI hallmark of ICC appeared to be, in fact, the presence of a progressive increase in enhancement or sustained enhancement in the portal/venous phases followed by an enhancement defect in the post-vascular phase. This differs slightly from the findings of Park et al. [44], who found 6 or 32 ICC nodules to show the typical HCC pattern (hyperenhancement followed by washout); however, it was not specified in their work whether these findings occurred in patients with or without cirrhosis, despite only half of their population having chronic liver disease with the usual etiologies. Second, these authors find a target appearance in the HB at 10 min in ICC, but much less at 20 min [44]. Thus, the latter appearance's was compared with our own ones, and indeed they were much in agreement. These findings, contributing to a correct suspicion upon ICC and an accurate distinction of ICC from HCC using MRI with hepatocyte-specific contrast agents support the choice of Japanese experts to recommend such a type of MRI for the recall strategy of patients with focal liver lesions in cirrhosis [20, 38], which had not yet been adopted by other societies [45].

Clearly, the present study has limitations. First is the absence of patients with decompensated liver disease with jaundice, therefore leaving unresolved the question whether the clinical stage of cirrhosis affects the diagnostic accuracy of MRI using a contrast agent that is specifically metabolized by liver cells. The uptake of EOB-Gd in cirrhosis decreases in fact with the deterioration of liver function [46]. Thus, the argument is that radiological confirmation of ICC could be challenged in cirrhotic patients with moderately or severely elevated bilirubin, a patient population that, however, is poorly represented in surveillance programs, since these patients are unsuitable to most therapies for liver cancer. In our study, all patients were in Child-Pugh class A with normal levels of bilirubin, like all patients enrolled in the previous study in Spain [2], a fact that further grants for the clinical relevance of the non-invasive diagnosis of ICC in compensated cirrhotics who are eligible to radical treatments. Another limitation is the small number of non-HCC lesions. In fact, these lesions were reported to incidentally show hyperintensity on delayed venous phase at MRI [5] and a few showed enhancement defect in the hepatobiliary phase in our study. Further larger studies on the latter type of lesions with special attention to the differential diagnosis with ICC rather than HCC are therefore recommended, but it has to be acknowledged that collecting such large prospective series of histologically confirmed lesions, investigated by MRI with hepatobiliary agents is quite difficult. In fact, since the rate of ICC in cirrhosis is reported to be around 1.5% of new nodules [6, 47, 48], the prospective collection of this same amount of histologically confirmed ICC lesions as in the present study (16 lesions) would have required about 1,000 patients with new nodules submitted to MRI and with subsequent biopsy. If the number of lesions to be collected is requested to be even larger than that of the present study, an enrollment of many thousands of patients submitted to MRI and histological confirmation would be necessary, which is hardly achievable even by multicentric studies.

In conclusion, MRI with hepatocyte-specific Gd-based contrast agents allows differentiating ICC from both regenerative and HCC nodules. In fact, during the vascular phases, the behavior of ICC is different from the typical HCC patter, while the hypointense pattern in the delayed phase differentiates ICC from those benign nodules that might have a similar pattern in the vascular phases.

Disclosure Statement

In connection with the present article we disclose that F. Piscaglia, M. Iavarone, A. Sangiovanni, R. Golfieri, M. Colombo and L. Bolondi have received advisory board and/or speaker fees from Bayer. F. Piscaglia and L. Bolondi have received speaker fees from Bracco.

References

1 Clinical practice guidelines for hepatocellular carcinoma differ between Japan, United States, and Europe. Liver Cancer 2015;4:85–95.

2 Rimola J, Forner A, Reig M, Vilana R, de Lope CR, Ayuso C, Bruix J: Cholangiocarcinoma in cirrhosis: absence of contrast washout in delayed phases by magnetic resonance imaging avoids misdiagnosis of hepatocellular carcinoma. Hepatology 2009;50:791–798.

3 Vilana R, Forner A, Bianchi L, García-Criado A, Rimola J, de Lope CR, Reig M, Ayuso C, Brú C, Bruix J: Intrahepatic peripheral cholangiocarcinoma in cirrhosis patients may display a vascular pattern similar to hepatocellular carcinoma on contrast-enhanced ultrasound. Hepatology 2010;51:2020–2029.

4 Boozari B, Soudah B, Rifai K, Schneidewind S, Vogel A, Hecker H, Hahn A, Schlue J, Dietrich CF, Bahr MJ, Kubicka S, Manns MP, Gebel M: Grading of hypervascular hepatocellular carcinoma using late phase of contrast enhanced sonography – a prospective study. Dig Liver Dis 2011;43:484–490.

5 Rimola J, Forner A, Tremosini S, Reig M, Vilana R, Bianchi L, Rodríguez-Lope C, Solé M, Ayuso C, Bruix J: Non-invasive diagnosis of hepatocellular carcinoma ≤2 cm in cirrhosis. Diagnostic accuracy assessing fat, capsule and signal intensity at dynamic MRI. J Hepatol 2012;56:1317–1323.

6 Sangiovanni A, Manini MA, Iavarone M, Romeo R, Forzenigo LV, Fraquelli M, Massironi S, Della Corte C, Ronchi G, Rumi MG, Biondetti P, Colombo M: The diagnostic and economic impact of contrast imaging techniques in the diagnosis of small hepatocellular carcinoma in cirrhosis. Gut 2010;59:638–644.
7 Serste T, Barrau V, Ozenne V, Vullierme MP, Bedossa P, Farges O, Valla DC, Vilgrain V, Paradis V, Degos F: Accuracy and disagreement of computed tomography and magnetic resonance imaging for the diagnosis of small hepatocellular carcinoma and dysplastic nodules: role of biopsy. Hepatology 2012;55:800–806.
8 Dietrich CF, Mertens JC, Braden B, Schuessler G, Ott M, Ignee A: Contrast-enhanced ultrasound of histologically proven liver hemangiomas. Hepatology 2007;45:1139–1145.
9 Leoni S, Piscaglia F, Golfieri R, Camaggi V, Vidili G, Pini P, Bolondi L: The impact of vascular and nonvascular findings on the noninvasive diagnosis of small hepatocellular carcinoma based on the EASL and AASLD criteria. Am J Gastroenterol 2010;105:599–609.
10 van Montfoort JE, Stieger B, Meijer DK, Weinmann HJ, Meier PJ, Fattinger KE: Hepatic uptake of the magnetic resonance imaging contrast agent gadoxetate by the organic anion transporting polypeptide Oatp1. J Pharmacol Exp Ther 1999;290:153–157.
11 Bartolozzi C, Crocetti L, Lencioni R, Cioni D, Della Pina C, Campani D: Biliary and reticuloendothelial impairment in hepatocarcinogenesis: the diagnostic role of tissue-specific MR contrast media. Eur Radiol 2007;17:2519–2530.
12 Giovagnoni A, Paci E: Liver. III: gadolinium-based hepatobiliary contrast agents (Gd-EOB-DTPA and Gd-BOPTA/Dimeg). Magn Reson Imaging Clin N Am 1996;4:61–72.
13 Ichikawa S, Ichikawa T, Motosugi U, Sano K, Morisaka H, Enomoto N: Was hypervascular hepatocellular carcinoma visible on previous gadoxetic acid-enhanced magnetic resonance images? Liver Cancer 2015;4:154–162.
14 Choi SH, Lee JM, Yu NC, Suh KS, Jang JJ, Kim SH, Choi BI: Hepatocellular carcinoma in liver transplantation candidates: detection with gadobenate dimeglumine-enhanced MRI. AJR Am J Roentgenol 2008;191:529–536.
15 Fidler J, Hough D: Hepatocyte-specific magnetic resonance imaging contrast agents. Hepatology 2011;53:678–682.
16 Jeong WK, Byun JH, Lee SS, Won HJ, Kim KW, Shin YM, Kim PN, Lee MG: Gadobenate dimeglumine-enhanced liver MR imaging in cirrhotic patients: quantitative and qualitative comparison of 1-hour and 3-hour delayed images. J Magn Reson Imaging 2011;33:889–897.
17 Lee JM, Zech CJ, Bolondi L, Jonas E, Kim MJ, Matsui O, Merkle EM, Sakamoto M, Choi BI: Consensus report of the 4th international forum for gadolinium-ethoxybenzyl-diethylenetriamine pentaacetic acid magnetic resonance imaging. Korean J Radiol 2011;12:403–415.
18 Saito K, Kotake F, Ito N, Ozuki T, Mikami R, Abe K, Shimazaki Y: Gd-EOB-DTPA enhanced MRI for hepatocellular carcinoma: quantitative evaluation of tumor enhancement in hepatobiliary phase. Magn Reson Med Sci 2005;4:1–9.
19 Golfieri R, Renzulli M, Lucidi V, Corcioni B, Trevisani F, Bolondi L: Contribution of the hepatobiliary phase of Gd-EOB-DTPA-enhanced MRI to dynamic MRI in the detection of hypovascular small (≤ 2 cm) HCC in cirrhosis. Eur Radiol 2011;21:1233–1242.
20 Kudo M, Izumi N, Kokudo N, Matsui O, Sakamoto M, Nakashima O, Kojiro M, Makuuchi M; HCC Expert Panel of Japan Society of Hepatology: Management of hepatocellular carcinoma in Japan: consensus-based clinical practice guidelines proposed by the Japan society of hepatology (JSH) 2010 updated version. Dig Dis 2011;29:339–364.
21 Kudo M, Matsui O, Izumi N, Iijima H, Kadoya M, Imai Y, Okusaka T, Miyayama S, Tsuchiya K, Ueshima K, Hiraoka A, Ikeda M, Ogasawara S, Yamashita T, Minami T, Yamakado K; Liver Cancer Study Group of Japan: JSH consensus-based clinical practice guidelines for the management of hepatocellular carcinoma: 2014 update by the Liver Cancer Study Group of Japan. Liver Cancer 2014;3:458–468.
22 Murakami T, Tsurusaki M: Hypervascular benign and malignant liver tumors that require differentiation from hepatocellular carcinoma: key points of imaging diagnosis. Liver Cancer 2014;3:85–96.
23 Chen LD, Xu HX, Xie XY, Xie XH, Xu ZF, Liu GJ, Wang Z, Lin MX, Lu MD: Intrahepatic cholangiocarcinoma and hepatocellular carcinoma: differential diagnosis with contrast-enhanced ultrasound. Eur Radiol 2010;20:743–753.
24 Claudon M, Dietrich CF, Choi BI, Cosgrove DO, Kudo M, Nolsøe CP, Piscaglia F, Wilson SR, Barr RG, Chammas MC, Chaubal NG, Chen MH, Clevert DA, Correas JM, Ding H, Forsberg F, Fowlkes JB, Gibson RN, Goldberg BB, Lassau N, Leen EL, Mattrey RF, Moriyasu F, Solbiati L, Weskott HP, Xu HX: Guidelines and good clinical practice recommendations for contrast enhanced ultrasound (CEUS) in the liver – update 2012: a WFUMB-EFSUMB initiative in cooperation with representatives of AFSUMB, AIUM, ASUM, FLAUS and ICUS. Ultraschall Med 2013;34:11–29.
25 Yuan MX, Li R, Zhang XH, Tang CL, Guo YL, Guo DY, Luo MK: Factors affecting the enhancement patterns of intrahepatic cholangiocarcinoma (ICC) on contrast-enhanced ultrasound (CEUS) and their pathological correlations in patients with a single lesion. Ultraschall Med 2015, Epub ahead of print, DOI: 10.1055/s-0034-1399485.
26 European Association for the Study of the Liver; European Organisation for Research and Treatment of Cancer: EASL-EORTC clinical practice guidelines: management of hepatocellular carcinoma. J Hepatol 2012;56:908–943.
27 Kokudo N, Hasegawa K, Akahane M, Igaki H, Izumi N, Ichida T, Uemoto S, Kaneko S, Kawasaki S, Ku Y, Kudo M, Kubo S, Takayama T, Tateishi R, Fukuda T, Matsui O, Matsuyama Y, Murakami T, Arii S, Okazaki M, Makuuchi M: Evidence-based clinical practice guidelines for hepatocellular carcinoma: the Japan society of hepatology 2013 update (3rd JSH-HCC guidelines). Hepatol Res 2015;45.
28 Chalasani N, Younossi Z, Lavine JE, Diehl AM, Brunt EM, Cusi K, Charlton M, Sanyal AJ: The diagnosis and management of non-alcoholic fatty liver disease: practice guideline by the American Association for the Study of Liver Diseases, American College of Gastroenterology, and the American Gastroenterological Association. Hepatology 2012;55:2005–2023.
29 Granito A, Galassi M, Piscaglia F, Romanini L, Lucidi V, Renzulli M, Borghi A, Grazioli L, Golfieri R, Bolondi L: Impact of gadoxetic acid (Gd-EOB-DTPA)-enhanced magnetic resonance on the non-invasive diagnosis of small hepatocellular carcinoma: a prospective study. Aliment Pharmacol Ther 2013;37:355–363.
30 Bruix J, Sherman M; American Association for the Study of Liver Diseases: Management of hepatocellular carcinoma: an update. Hepatology 2011;53:1020–1022.
31 Morana G, Grazioli L, Kirchin MA, Bondioni MP, Faccioli N, Guarise A, Schneider G: Solid hypervascular liver lesions: accurate identification of true benign lesions on enhanced dynamic and hepatobiliary phase magnetic resonance imaging after gadobenate dimeglumine administration. Invest Radiol 2011;46:225–239.
32 Harris MA, Johnson TR, Weinberg PM, Fogel MA: Delayed-enhancement cardiovascular magnetic resonance identifies fibrous tissue in children after surgery for congenital heart disease. J Thorac Cardiovasc Surg 2007;133:676–681.
33 Kramer CM, Cerilli LA, Hagspiel K, DiMaria JM, Epstein FH, Kern JA: Magnetic resonance imaging identifies the fibrous cap in atherosclerotic abdominal aortic aneurysm. Circulation 2004;109:1016–1021.
34 Ahn SS, Kim MJ, Lim JS, Hong HS, Chung YE, Choi JY: Added value of gadoxetic acid-enhanced hepatobiliary phase MR imaging in the diagnosis of hepatocellular carcinoma. Radiology 2010;255:459–466.
35 Piscaglia F, Bolondi L: Recent advances in the diagnosis of hepatocellular carcinoma. Hepatol Res 2007;37(suppl 2):S178–S192.
36 Ichikawa T, Sano K, Morisaka H: Diagnosis of pathologically early HCC with EOB-MRI: experiences and current consensus. Liver Cancer 2014;3:97–107.
37 Kudo M: Early hepatocellular carcinoma: definition and diagnosis. Liver Cancer 2013;2:69–72.

38 Kudo M, Matsui O, Izumi N, Iijima H, Kadoya M, Imai Y; Liver Cancer Study Group of Japan: Surveillance and diagnostic algorithm for hepatocellular carcinoma proposed by the Liver Cancer Study Group of Japan: 2014 update. Oncology 2014;87(suppl 1):7–21.
39 Lee JI, Campbell JS: Role of desmoplasia in cholangiocarcinoma and hepatocellular carcinoma. J Hepatol 2014;61:432–434.
40 Doo KW, Lee CH, Choi JW, Lee J, Kim KA, Park CM: 'Pseudo washout' sign in high-flow hepatic hemangioma on gadoxetic acid contrast-enhanced MRI mimicking hypervascular tumor. AJR Am J Roentgenol 2009; 193:W490–W496.
41 Fowler KJ, Brown JJ, Narra VR: Magnetic resonance imaging of focal liver lesions: approach to imaging diagnosis. Hepatology 2011;54:2227–2237.
42 Ahn SJ, Kim MJ, Hong HS, Kim KA, Song HT: Distinguishing hemangiomas from malignant solid hepatic lesions: a comparison of heavily T2-weighted images obtained before and after administration of gadoxetic acid. J Magn Reson Imaging 2011;34:310–317.
43 Tamada T, Ito K, Yamamoto A, Sone T, Kanki A, Tanaka F, Higashi H: Hepatic hemangiomas: evaluation of enhancement patterns at dynamic MRI with gadoxetate disodium. AJR Am J Roentgenol 2011;196:824–830.
44 Park HJ, Kim YK, Park MJ, Lee WJ: Small intrahepatic mass-forming cholangiocarcinoma: target sign on diffusion-weighted imaging for differentiation from hepatocellular carcinoma. Abdom Imaging 2013;38:793–801.
45 Bota S, Piscaglia F, Marinelli S, Pecorelli A, Terzi E, Bolondi L: Comparison of international guidelines for noninvasive diagnosis of hepatocellular carcinoma. Liver Cancer 2012; 1:190–200.
46 Hsu C, Chen BB, Chen CH, Ho MC, Cheng JC, Kokudo N, Murakami T, Yeo W, Seong J, Jia JD, Han KH, Cheng AL: Consensus development from the 5th Asia-Pacific Primary Liver Cancer Expert Meeting (APPLE 2014). Liver Cancer 2015;4:96–105.
47 Forner A, Vilana R, Ayuso C, Bianchi L, Solé M, Ayuso JR, Boix L, Sala M, Varela M, Llovet JM, Brú C, Bruix J: Diagnosis of hepatic nodules 20 mm or smaller in cirrhosis: prospective validation of the noninvasive diagnostic criteria for hepatocellular carcinoma. Hepatology 2008;47:97–104.
48 Leoni S, Piscaglia F, Granito A, Borghi A, Galassi M, Marinelli S, Terzi E, Bolondi L: Characterization of primary and recurrent nodules in liver cirrhosis using contrast-enhanced ultrasound: which vascular criteria should be adopted? Ultraschall Med 2013;34: 280–287.

Original Article

Digestive Diseases

Dig Dis 2015;33:745–750
DOI: 10.1159/000439098

Hepatic DNA Methylation Is Affected by Hepatocellular Carcinoma Risk in Patients with and without Hepatitis Virus

Naoshi Nishida Mina Iwanishi Tomohiro Minami Hirokazu Chishina Tadaaki Arizumi Masahiro Takita Satoshi Kitai Norihisa Yada Hiroshi Ida Satoru Hagiwara Yasunori Minami Kazuomi Ueshima Toshiharu Sakurai Masayuki Kitano Masatoshi Kudo

Department of Gastroenterology and Hepatology, Kinki University School of Medicine, Osaka-Sayama, Osaka, Japan

Key Words

DNA methylation · Hepatocellular carcinoma · Background liver · Aging · Diabetes mellitus

Abstract

Objectives: Several studies revealed that the proportion of hepatocellular carcinoma (HCC) without hepatitis virus infection (NBNC-HCC) is increasing. On the other hand, epigenetic alterations are reportedly responsible for HCC development. Here, we identified HCC risk factors that are associated with DNA methylation in the background liver tissue of NBNC-HCC patients. ***Methods:*** We performed methylation analysis in 37 pairs of virus-positive and 22 pairs of NBNC-HCC and non-cancerous livers using a HumanMethylation450 BeadChip array. After the selection of differentially methylated CpGs (DM-CpGs) in cancerous and non-cancerous livers, we analyzed DNA methylation of DM-CpGs within the adjacent non-cancerous liver tissue that is affected by specific HCC risk factors. ***Results:*** A total of 38,331 CpGs were selected as DM-CpGs using the following criteria: difference of β-value between HCC and non-cancerous liver ≥0.15 and false discovery rate (FDR) q < 1.0E-12. We subsequently selected the DM-CpGs that had methylation differences with the background liver tissue (that has FDR q < 0.35). Among the virus-positive patients, the type of hepatitis virus was mostly associated with differences in methylation within the background liver tissues. However, we found that background methylation patterns were most significantly associated with aging in NBNC patients. Interestingly, age-related methylation differences in DM-CpGs were also observed in NBNC-HCC tissues. ***Conclusions:*** Hepatitis viruses affect the methylation profiles within background liver tissues. However, difference in background methylation was mostly associated with age in NCBC-HCC patients; some age-related methylation events could contribute to emergence of NBNC-HCC in elderly individuals.

Introduction

Hepatitis B virus (HBV) and hepatitis C virus (HCV) infections are the best known causes of hepatocellular carcinoma (HCC), so far [1, 2]. Therefore, recent development of antiviral therapy was aimed at decreasing the

KARGER 125

E-Mail karger@karger.com
www.karger.com/ddi

Naoshi Nishida, MD
Department of Gastroenterology and Hepatology
Kinki University School of Medicine
337-2 Ohno-Higashi, Osaka-Sayama, Osaka 589-8511 (Japan)
E-Mail naoshi@med.kindai.ac.jp

incidence of hepatitis virus-related HCCs [3]. However, several studies revealed that the proportion of HCC patients, which are not related to HBV and HCV infections (NBNC-HCC), is increasing especially in elderly patients [4, 5]. It is well documented that life style contributes to NBNC-HCC emergence, such as alcohol intake, increased prevalence of non-alcoholic fatty liver disease (NAFLD), diabetes mellitus and aging [6, 7].

Recent comprehensive analyses revealed that many kinds of genetic and epigenetic alterations were observed in background liver and HCC tissues [8, 9]. Therefore, it is conceivable that hepatocytes with genetic and epigenetic alterations in non-cancerous livers could act as a 'seed' for HCC emergence. Previously, we reported that number of methylated tumor suppressor genes was associated with time to HCC emergence in chronic hepatitis C patients [10]. This evidence also supported the idea that the degree of epigenetic alterations in chronic hepatitis should be an HCC development risk [11]. It has also been reported that oxidative DNA damage could induce epigenetic alterations that might be critical for hepatocarcinogenesis [12–14]; the known risks of NBNC-HCC, such as alcohol intake and the presence of NAFLD, could induce oxidative stress in hepatocytes [15]. This, in turn, can induce specific epigenetic alterations that are responsible for hepatocarcinogenesis [16, 17]. In this study, we attempted to identify a known HCC risk factor that is associated with DNA methylation in the background liver of NBNC-HCC patients. More specifically, we selected the differentially methylated CpGs (DM-CpGs) loci in HCC and non-cancerous background liver (DM-CpGs). Subsequently, we analyzed the differences in methylation of DM-CpGs in the context of specific risks for NBNC-HCCs and virus-related HCCs. We identified risk factors that were associated with unique HCC-related methylation events in NBNC-HCC background liver.

Materials and Methods

Patients

We performed comprehensive methylation analysis on 22 pairs of cancerous and non-cancerous livers from the NBNC-HCC patients. Similarly, we analyzed hepatic methylation profiles in 37 pairs of cancerous and non-cancerous livers from the hepatitis virus-positive HCC patients.

The NBNC-HCC patients had a median age of 72 years (distribution 61–79); 15 were men and 7 were women. The median body mass index (BMI) was 23.5 (distribution 14.6–32.5). Ten of the 22 patients were diabetic, and 4 had cirrhotic whereas 14 had non-cirrhotic background liver tissues. Three HCCs were well-differentiated and 19 were moderately/poorly differentiated. Eight patients were alcoholics (intake >30 g/day for males and >20 g/day for females), whereas 14 were not. Of the 14 non-alcoholic patients, 7 had ballooning accompanied by steatosis in the background liver, which indicates the presence of non-alcoholic steatohepatitis.

The hepatitis virus-positive HCC patients had a median age of 61 years (distribution 42–75), and 25 were men whereas 14 were women. The median BMI was 23.8 (distribution 18.9–33.5). The diabetic status was not determined for 20 patients; of the other 17 patients, 2 were diabetic. Thirty-one had cirrhotic and 8 had non-cirrhotic background liver. Sixteen HCCs were well-differentiated and 23 were moderately/poorly-differentiated. Sixteen patients were positive for the HBV surface antigen, and 23 were positive for HCV antibody.

Selection of DM-CpGs between Cancerous and Non-Cancerous Liver

For comprehensive methylation analyses, we used the Illumina Infinium HumanMethylation450 BeadChip array (Illumina, Inc., San Diego, Calif., USA). Among the 485,512 probes covering 99% of NCBI reference sequence database genes, we eliminated the probes that contained single-nucleotide polymorphisms or those located on sex chromosomes. Details of the methylation analysis using the HumanMethylation450 BeadChip were published previously [18, 19]. DM-CpG selection was performed if there was a difference in β-value between the cancerous and noncancerous liver ≥0.15 and false discovery rate (FDR) q-value using the Benjamini–Hochberg procedure <1.0E-12. Consequently, 38,331 CpGs that met these criteria were considered DM-CpGs.

DM-CpGs in Background Liver Tissues and Specific HCC Risk Factors

Among the 38,331 DM-CpGs described above, methylation profile differences based on HCC risk factors were also explored in adjacent non-cancerous livers. For this purpose, we further selected DM-CpGs between background livers with and without specific HCC risk factors; we analyzed methylation differences within the liver tissues between HBV surface antigen- and HCV antibody-positive patients in the virus-related HCC group. Similarly, we analyzed methylation differences between cirrhotic and non-cirrhotic, male and female as well as elderly (≥70 years) and non-elderly (≤69 years) livers in the virus-positive group. For the NBNC-HCC group, we analyzed methylation differences between habitual drinker and non-drinker, diabetic and non-diabetic, cirrhotic and non-cirrhotic, elderly and non-elderly, male and female and obese (BMI ≥25) and non-obese (BMI <25) livers. DM-CpGs with methylation differences within the background liver with FDR q-value <0.35 were selected as risk factor-specific CpGs.

Statistics

The Mann–Whitney U test and the FDR control using the Benjamini–Hochberg procedure were applied for multiple comparisons. The Pearson's chi-square test or the Fisher's exact test was used to compare categorical variables. Principle component analysis and hierarchical clustering analysis were performed to categorize the tissues based on methylation levels. All statistical analyses were conducted using the program R-3.0.3 (www.r-project.org) and JMP version 9.0 software (SAS Institute Inc., Cary, N.C., USA).

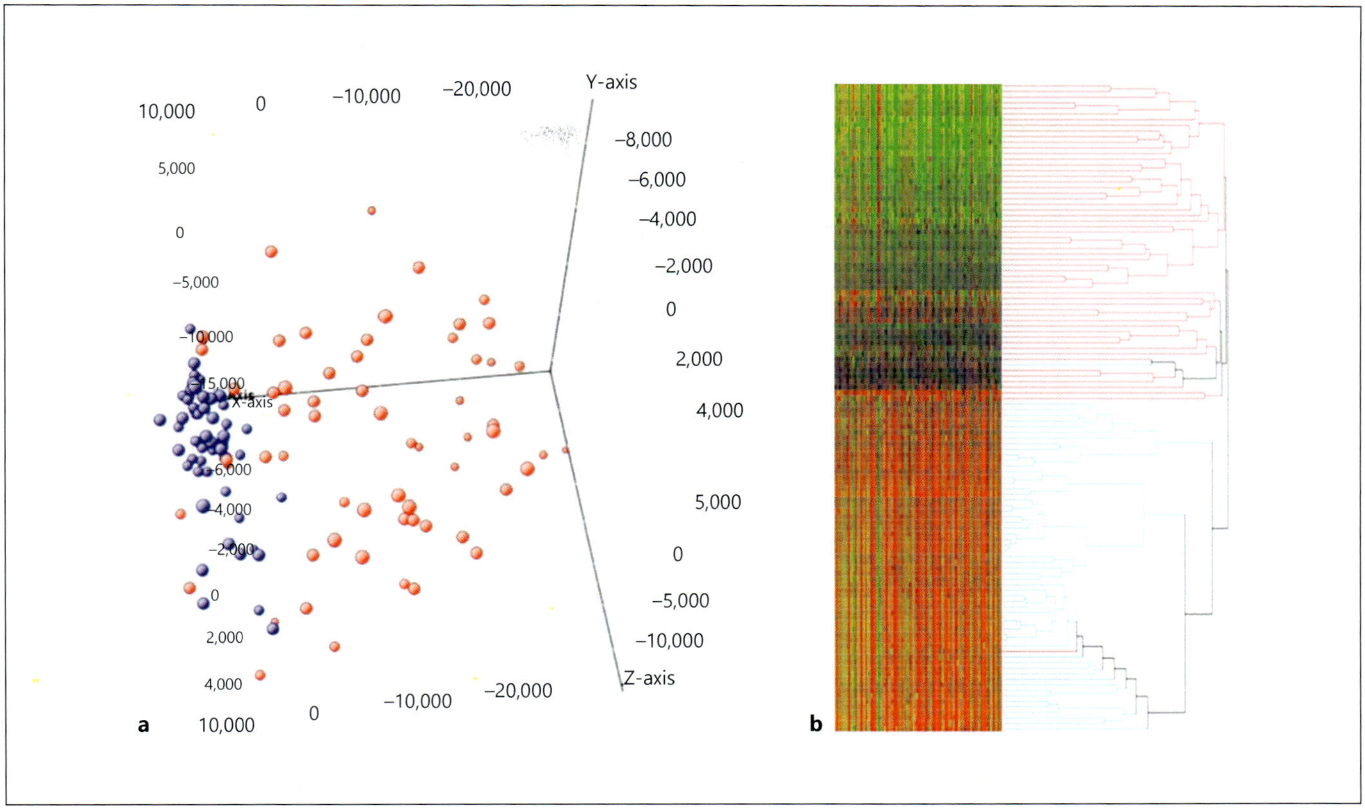

Fig. 1. Discrimination of cancerous and non-cancerous tissue using DNA methylation. **a** Principle component analysis using β-values of top 500 DM-CpGs that were most differently methylated between HCCs and non-cancerous livers. The red circle represents cancerous and the blue circle shows non-cancerous liver tissues. The methylation events are much more homogeneous in non-cancerous livers than in HCCs. **b** Hierarchical clustering analysis using β-values of top 500 DM-CpGs that are most differently methylated between HCCs and non-cancerous livers. All but 1 HCC are clearly discriminated from non-cancerous livers. The red lines and blue lines represent HCCs and non-cancerous livers, respectively.

Results

DM-CpGs between Cancerous and Non-Cancerous Liver

As described above, we selected 38,331 DM-CpGs. Of these, 3,052 showed increased methylation in HCC tissues, and 35,279 DM-CpGs had decreased methylation in HCC. We performed principle component analysis using β-values of the top 500 DM-CpGs that were most differentially methylated in the cancerous and non-cancerous livers (fig. 1a). The HCC tissues had a more scattered distribution than non-cancerous liver tissues, which indicates heterogeneity of methylation profiles in HCC tissues; methylation was homogeneous in non-cancerous livers compared to that of HCCs. HCC tissues were also clearly differentiated from non-cancerous liver using β-values of the top 500 DM-CpGs by hierarchical clustering analysis (fig. 1b).

Risk Factor-Specific DM-CpGs within the Background Liver of Virus-Positive and NBNC-HCC Patients

We selected the risk factor-specific DM-CpGs within the background liver of both hepatitis virus-positive and NBNC-HCC patients as described in the Materials and Methods. In hepatitis virus-positive HCC group, 11,164 of the 38,331 DM-CpGs (29%) were selected as risk factor-specific DM-CpGs between HBV- and HCV-positive background livers and were considered virus-related DM-CpGs. Similarly, we found that 2,896 DM-CpGs were associated with the presence of cirrhosis (cirrhosis-related DM-CpGs), and 1,164 were sex-related DM-CpGs. However, no DM-CpGs were selected between elderly and non-elderly background liver. On the contrary, within the non-cancerous livers of the NBNC-HCC patients, the risk factor most significantly associated with difference of methylation level were aging, 6,517 of 38,331 DM-CpGs (17%) were selected as age-

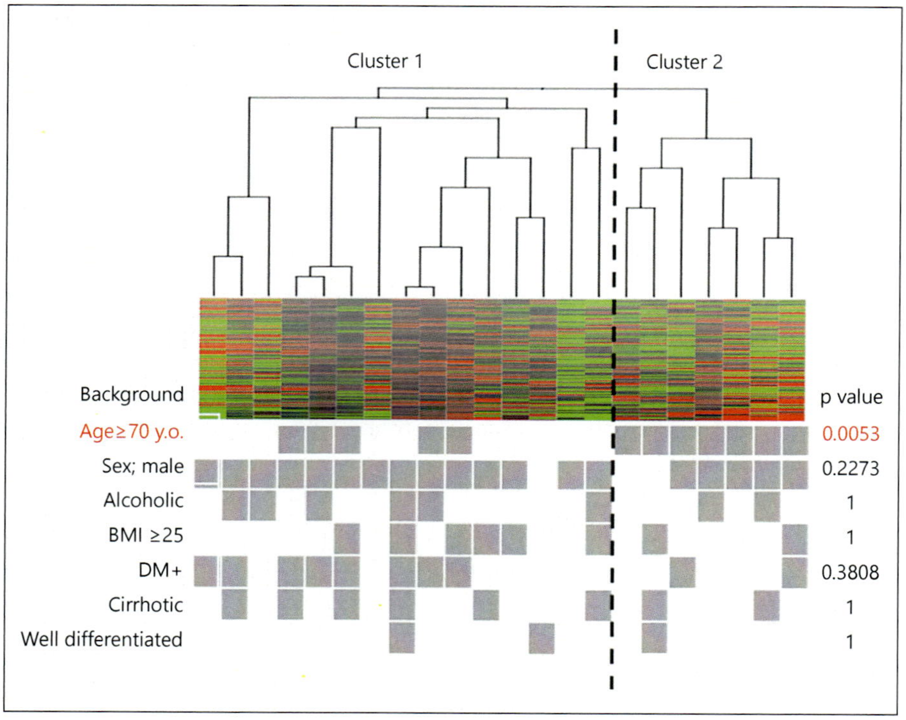

Fig. 2. Classification of HCC using methylation level of age-related DM-CpGs. The hierarchical clustering analysis based on the β-values of these top 340 age-related DM-CpGs quantified in HCC tissues. HCCs are successfully classified into 2 subgroups according to the β-values of 340 age-related DM-CpGs. Among the 15 HCCs that are classified into cluster 1, 10 are from the non-elderly (≤69 years) and 5 are from the elderly (≥70 years). On the other hand, all 7 HCCs classified into cluster 2 are members of the elderly group. The gray square represents the HCCs with specific risk factors or differentiation. p values by the Fisher's exact test are shown.

related DM-CpGs between elderly and non-elderly background liver, followed by the presence of diabetes mellitus, 47 DM-CpGs were diabetes-related risk factors (diabetes-related DM-CpGs). On the other hand, none of the methylation events on the DM-CpGs were affected by the presence or absence of cirrhosis, difference of sex or BMI. Interestingly, we could not find any DM-CpGs between alcoholic and non-alcoholic background liver.

Age-Related Methylation within Background Liver Could Affect NBNC-HCC Methylation Patterns

Among the 6,517 age-related DM-CpGs in background liver, 340 had β-values ≥0.15 between elderly and non-elderly livers. We classified tumors by hierarchical clustering analysis based on the β-values of the top 340 age-related DM-CpGs quantified in HCC tissues. We successfully classified HCCs into 2 subgroups (fig. 2); all HCCs that belonged to cluster 2 emerged from elderly patients ($p = 0.0053$ by the Fisher's exact test). Alternatively, other parameters, such as sex, alcohol intake, BMI, presence of DM, cirrhosis and tumor differentiation, did not affect this classification, which indicates that the methylation status of age-related DM-CpGs in NBNC-HCC tissues could be specifically affected by that of the background liver in elderly patients.

Discussion

Although the overall prevalence of the at-risk population for HCC is still growing, there is a recent trend showing an increase in proportion of NBNC-HCC patients in Japan [1, 5]. There are several risks for developing NBNC-HCC such as alcohol consumption, aging, presence of diabetes mellitus, obesity and hepatic iron overload [20]; some of these could act in concert and contribute to carcinogenesis.

On the other hand, several reports described epigenetic alterations in HCCs [21–23]; these molecular events could be, at least partially, attributed to the induction of oxidative DNA in the damaged hepatocytes. Previously, we reported that oxidative DNA damage could induce abnormal DNA methylation that is associated with HCC emergence [14]. Based on this background, we examined the difference of methylation profiles in the background liver of the HCC patients in the context of specific risks for HCC emergence that was associated with the oxidative stress.

First, we selected the CpGs that showed methylation differences between cancerous and non-cancerous liver (DM-CpGs) based on the β-value obtained from Human-Methylation450 BeadChip array analysis that reflected the methylation level of CpGs. As previously described, methylation events in the selected 38,331 DM-CpGs loci should represent the unique pattern of HCC-related DNA methylation alterations. Alternatively, it may be possible that some HCC risks might affect the methylation profile within background liver; some of these background alterations should contribute to hepatocarcinogenesis through the 'epigenetic pathway'.

Then, we attempted to clarify which risks could affect the methylation differences of the DM-CpGs within the background liver. Among the virus-positive patients, the type of hepatitis virus (HBV vs. HCV) was most associated with methylation difference in DM-CpGs. Previously, several reports showed the difference of methylation profiles between HBV- and HCV-related HCCs [24]. We also reported methylation differences within the non-cancerous livers of HBV- and HCV-positive patients [8, 25]. Integration of HBV into the host genome is a possible major mechanism of HCC emergence in HBV-related carcinogenesis [26], but this should not be the case in HCV-related HCCs. Therefore, disturbance of the host genome, but not DNA methylation, might be more important in a subset of HBV- than that of HCV-related carcinogenesis. In addition, integration of HBV that could trigger the DNA methylation at flanking genomic sequences should give rise to the methylation difference between HBV- and HCV-positive livers [27].

Our analysis also revealed that the degree of background fibrosis is associated with methylation difference. In the virus-related HCC group, liver fibrosis was more prominent in HCV- than in HBV-positive patients; this might lead to methylation status differences of DM-CpGs between cirrhotic and non-cirrhotic livers [28]. Alternatively, the duration of hepatitis, which should be related fibrosis progression, could affect DM-CpG loci methylation within the background liver. We also found that DM-CpG methylation patterns in background liver were most significantly associated with aging in NBNC patients, followed by the presence or the absence of diabetes mellitus, whereas fibrosis, alcohol intake and degree of BMI did not affect background methylation difference. Previous studies suggested that fibrosis and alcohol intake could affect DNA methylation of the liver tissues [29, 30]. Due to obesity as well as alcohol intake, NAFLD could increase oxidative stress and DNA damage in hepatocytes; therefore, it is conceivable that both NAFLD and alcohol intake might contribute to hepatocarcinogenesis via the same epigenetic pathway, which would lead to a lack of difference in the methylation profile within the background liver tissues, regardless of the fibrosis stage.

We found a large number of DM-CpGs between elderly and non-elderly livers in NBNC group. Therefore, aging may affect the DNA methylation in the background liver, which has also been previously reported. In addition, these age-related DM-CpGs methylation in NBNC patients were also observed in HCC tissues. This evidence also supports the idea that methylation events that emerge during the aging process might play a role in HCC development [31], and clonal expansion of hepatocytes with age-related methylation could take place. The specific age-related methylation events that could drive carcinogenesis in virus-negative patients are currently under investigation.

In this report, we showed that the type of hepatitis virus affected the methylation profile in the background liver of HBV- and HCV-related HCC patients. However, methylation difference within the background liver was most prominent between elderly and non-elderly NCBC-HCC patients; some of these methylation events could contribute to emergence of NBNC-HCC. Further studies are necessary to elucidate the role of age-related epigenetic alteration on NBNC-HCC emergence.

Acknowledgments

This work was supported in part by Grant-in-Aid for Scientific Research (KAKENHI: 24590997) from the Japanese Society for the Promotion of Science (N. Nishida), a grant from the Smoking Research Foundation (N. Nishida) and a grant from the Japan Health Foundation (N. Nishida).

Disclosure Statement

The authors have no conflicts of interest to disclose.

References

1 Kudo M: Surveillance, diagnosis, treatment, and outcome of liver cancer in Japan. Liver Cancer 2015;4:39–50.
2 Kawanaka M, Nishino K, Nakamura J, Oka T, Urata N, Goto D, Suehiro M, Kawamoto H, Kudo M, Yamada G: Quantitative levels of hepatitis B virus DNA and surface antigen and the risk of hepatocellular carcinoma in patients with hepatitis B receiving long-term nucleos(t)ide analogue therapy. Liver Cancer 2014;3:41–52.
3 Webster DP, Klenerman P, Dusheiko GM: Hepatitis C. Lancet 2015;385:1124–1135.
4 Kudo M: Treatment of advanced hepatocellular carcinoma with emphasis on hepatic arterial infusion chemotherapy and molecular targeted therapy. Liver Cancer 2012;1:62–70.

5 Tateishi R, Okanoue T, Fujiwara N, Okita K, Kiyosawa K, Omata M, Kumada H, Hayashi N, Koike K: Clinical characteristics, treatment, and prognosis of non-B, non-C hepatocellular carcinoma: a large retrospective multicenter cohort study. J Gastroenterol 2015; 50:350–360.
6 Honda T, Miyaaki H, Ichikawa T, Taura N, Miuma S, Shibata H, Isomoto H, Takeshima F, Nakao K: Clinical characteristics of hepatocellular carcinoma in elderly patients. Oncol Lett 2011;2:851–854.
7 Michelotti GA, Machado MV, Diehl AM: NAFLD, NASH and liver cancer. Nat Rev Gastroenterol Hepatol 2013;10:656–665.
8 Nishida N, Nagasaka T, Nishimura T, Ikai I, Boland CR, Goel A: Aberrant methylation of multiple tumor suppressor genes in aging liver, chronic hepatitis, and hepatocellular carcinoma. Hepatology 2008;47:908–918.
9 Nishida N, Kudo M: Recent advancements in comprehensive genetic analyses for human hepatocellular carcinoma. Oncology 2013; 84(suppl 1):93–97.
10 Nishida N, Kudo M, Nagasaka T, Ikai I, Goel A: Characteristic patterns of altered DNA methylation predict emergence of human hepatocellular carcinoma. Hepatology 2012;56: 994–1003.
11 Nishida N, Kudo M: Alteration of epigenetic profile in human hepatocellular carcinoma and its clinical implications. Liver Cancer 2014;3:417–427.
12 Lim SO, Gu JM, Kim MS, Kim HS, Park YN, Park CK, Cho JW, Park YM, Jung G: Epigenetic changes induced by reactive oxygen species in hepatocellular carcinoma: methylation of the E-cadherin promoter. Gastroenterology 2008;135:2128–2140, 2140.e1–e8.
13 O'Hagan HM, Wang W, Sen S, Destefano Shields C, Lee SS, Zhang YW, Clements EG, Cai Y, Van Neste L, Easwaran H, Casero RA, Sears CL, Baylin SB: Oxidative damage targets complexes containing DNA methyltransferases, SIRT1, and polycomb members to promoter CpG Islands. Cancer Cell 2011;20:606–619.
14 Nishida N, Arizumi T, Takita M, Kitai S, Yada N, Hagiwara S, Inoue T, Minami Y, Ueshima K, Sakurai T, Kudo M: Reactive oxygen species induce epigenetic instability through the formation of 8-hydroxydeoxyguanosine in human hepatocarcinogenesis. Dig Dis 2013; 31:459–466.
15 Bonomini F, Rodella LF, Rezzani R: Metabolic syndrome, aging and involvement of oxidative stress. Aging Dis 2015;6:109–120.
16 Nishida N, Kudo M: Oxidative stress and epigenetic instability in human hepatocarcinogenesis. Dig Dis 2013;31:447–453.
17 Szabo G, Petrasek J: Inflammasome activation and function in liver disease. Nat Rev Gastroenterol Hepatol 2015;12:387–400.
18 Shen J, Wang S, Zhang YJ, Wu HC, Kibriya MG, Jasmine F, Ahsan H, Wu DP, Siegel AB, Remotti H, Santella RM: Exploring genome-wide DNA methylation profiles altered in hepatocellular carcinoma using infinium HumanMethylation 450 BeadChips. Epigenetics 2013;8:34–43.
19 Nishida N, Nishimura T, Nakai T, Chishina H, Arizumi T, Takita M, Kitai S, Yada N, Hagiwara S, Inoue T, Minami Y, Ueshima K, Sakurai T, Kudo M: Genome-wide profiling of DNA methylation and tumor progression in human hepatocellular carcinoma. Dig Dis 2014;32:658–663.
20 Kew MC: Hepatic iron overload and hepatocellular carcinoma. Liver Cancer 2014;3:31–40.
21 Nishida N, Nishimura T, Nagasaka T, Ikai I, Goel A, Boland CR: Extensive methylation is associated with beta-catenin mutations in hepatocellular carcinoma: evidence for two distinct pathways of human hepatocarcinogenesis. Cancer Res 2007;67:4586–4594.
22 Nishida N, Goel A: Genetic and epigenetic signatures in human hepatocellular carcinoma: a systematic review. Curr Genomics 2011; 12:130–137.
23 Nishida N, Chishina H, Arizumi T, Takita M, Kitai S, Yada N, Hagiwara S, Inoue T, Minami Y, Ueshima K, Sakurai T, Kudo M: Identification of epigenetically inactivated genes in human hepatocellular carcinoma by integrative analyses of methylation profiling and pharmacological unmasking. Dig Dis 2014;32: 740–746.
24 Rongrui L, Na H, Zongfang L, Fanpu J, Shiwen J: Epigenetic mechanism involved in the HBV/HCV-related hepatocellular carcinoma tumorigenesis. Curr Pharm Des 2014;20: 1715–1725.
25 Nishida N, Kudo M, Nishimura T, Arizumi T, Takita M, Kitai S, Yada N, Hagiwara S, Inoue T, Minami Y, Ueshima K, Sakurai T, Yokomichi N, Nagasaka T, Goel A: Unique association between global DNA hypomethylation and chromosomal alterations in human hepatocellular carcinoma. PLoS One 2013; 8:e72312.
26 Shibata T, Aburatani H: Exploration of liver cancer genomes. Nat Rev Gastroenterol Hepatol 2014;11:340–349.
27 Watanabe Y, Yamamoto H, Oikawa R, Toyota M, Yamamoto M, Kokudo N, Tanaka S, Arii S, Yotsuyanagi H, Koike K, Itoh F: DNA methylation at hepatitis B viral integrants is associated with methylation at flanking human genomic sequences. Genome Res 2015; 25:328–337.
28 Mann DA: Epigenetics in liver disease. Hepatology 2014;60:1418–1425.
29 Murphy SK, Yang H, Moylan CA, Pang H, Dellinger A, Abdelmalek MF, Garrett ME, Ashley-Koch A, Suzuki A, Tillmann HL, Hauser MA, Diehl AM: Relationship between methylome and transcriptome in patients with nonalcoholic fatty liver disease. Gastroenterology 2013;145:1076–1087.
30 Zeybel M, Hardy T, Robinson SM, Fox C, Anstee QM, Ness T, Masson S, Mathers JC, French J, White S, Mann J: Differential DNA methylation of genes involved in fibrosis progression in non-alcoholic fatty liver disease and alcoholic liver disease. Clin Epigenetics 2015;7:25.
31 Herceg Z, Paliwal A: Epigenetic mechanisms in hepatocellular carcinoma: how environmental factors influence the epigenome. Mutat Res 2011;727:55–61.

Review Article

Digestive Diseases

Dig Dis 2015;33:751–758
DOI: 10.1159/000439290

Subclassification of BCLC B Stage Hepatocellular Carcinoma and Treatment Strategies: Proposal of Modified Bolondi's Subclassification (Kinki Criteria)

Masatoshi Kudo Tadaaki Arizumi Kazuomi Ueshima Toshiharu Sakurai Masayuki Kitano Naoshi Nishida

Department of Gastroenterology and Hepatology, Kinki University School of Medicine, Osaka-Sayama, Osaka, Japan

Key Words

BCLC staging · Intermediate stage · Hepatocellular carcinoma · Transarterial chemoembolization

Abstract

Intermediate stage hepatocellular carcinoma (HCC) is a very heterogeneous tumor in terms of tumor size (>3 cm ~ over 10 cm), tumor number (4 ~ over 20) and liver function (Child-Pugh score 5–9). However, transarterial chemoembolization is the only recommended treatment option according to the Barcelona Clinic Liver Cancer (BCLC) staging. Bolondi's subclassification of BCLC B stage is feasible; however, there are several weak points. Therefore, by modifying Bolondi's subclassification, we have proposed a more simplified subclassification, Kinki criteria. The Kinki criteria consist of 2 factors: liver function (Child-Pugh score 5–7 or 8, 9) and tumor status (Beyond Milan and within up-to-7 criteria; IN and OUT). The Kinki criteria classifies BCLC B stage from B1 (Child-Pugh score 5–7 and within up-to-7), B2 (Child-Pugh score 5–7 and beyond up-to-7) and B3 (Child-Pugh score 8, 9 and any tumor status). These criteria are simple and easy to apply to clinical practice. Therefore, these criteria will stratify the heterogeneous population of BCLC B group patient well and give the treatment indication according to each substage. These criteria should be further validated both retrospectively and prospectively.

Introduction

The Barcelona Clinic Liver Cancer (BCLC) group defines intermediate-stage hepatocellular carcinoma (HCC) as BCLC stage B. The BCLC staging system is applied in the guidelines published by the American Association for the Study of Liver Diseases (AASLD) [1] and the guidelines published collaboratively by the European Association for the Study of the Liver and the European Organization for Research and Treatment of Cancer [2]. However, the concept of intermediate-stage HCC is absent from the Japanese Evidence-based Clinical Practice Guidelines for Hepatocellular Carcinoma [3], the Consensus-based Clinical Practice Guideline for the Management of Hepatocellular Carcinoma [4, 5] and the guidelines published by the Asian Pacific Association for the Study of the Liver (APASL) [6]. If we consider the concept of intermediate-stage HCC for Japanese patients, patients with Child-Pugh grade A or B liver function and tumor size >3 cm or number of tumor >3 nodules and no vascular invasion or extrahepatic spread are included. In the BCLC staging system, only transarterial chemoembolization (TACE) is indicated for intermediate-stage HCC [7, 8] (fig. 1). However, the clinical manifestations of intermediate-stage HCC range extensively from those observed in patients with near early-stage HCC (who are candidates for curative treatment) to those observed in patients with near end-stage HCC

KARGER 125

E-Mail karger@karger.com
www.karger.com/ddi

Masatoshi Kudo, MD, PhD
Department of Gastroenterology and Hepatology
Kinki University School of Medicine, 377-2 Ohno-Higashi
Osaka-Sayama, Osaka 589-8511 (Japan)
E-Mail m-kudo@med.kindai.ac.jp

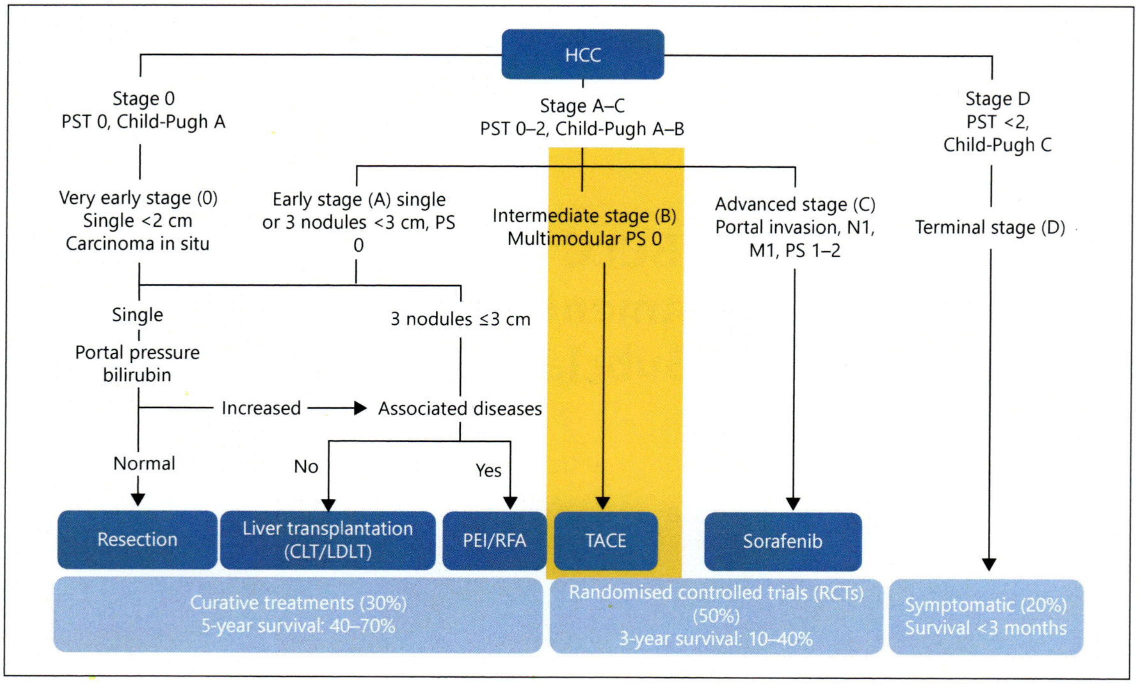

Fig. 1. Proposed AASLD-JNCI modification of BCLC staging: unresectable HCC.

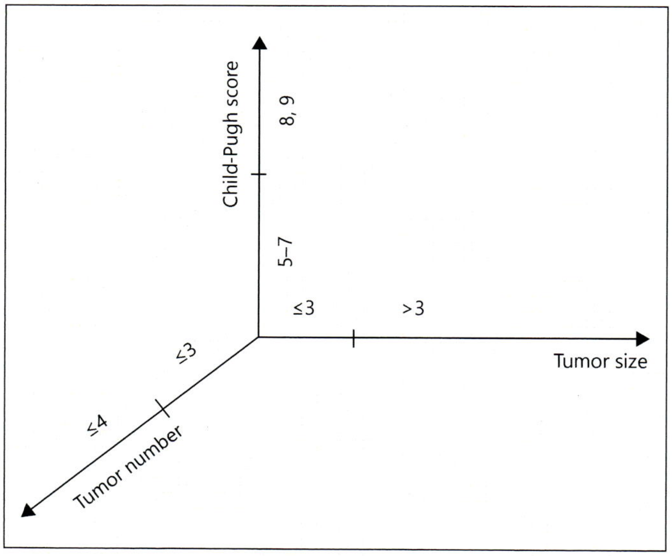

Fig. 2. Three dimensional factors (size, number and CP score) complicate subclassification of BCLC-B stage.

Table 1. Heterogeneity of intermediate-stage HCC

Liver function	Child-Pugh score 5–9
Tumor size	>5 cm ~ over 10 cm
Tumor number	≥4 ~ over 20 nodules

(Child-Pugh score of 9 who are candidates for best supportive care (BSC)).

In other words, BCLC staging indicates that intermediate-stage HCC should be treated only by TACE. However, in the real clinical setting, it is not always the case because of its heterogeneity in terms of liver function and/or tumor status. Therefore, subclassification of this heterogeneous patient population and indication of treatment strategy according to its substage is an extremely important issue to address.

Heterogeneity of Intermediate-Stage HCCs

BCLC stage B ranges from Child-Pugh scores 5–9 and thus includes an extremely large patient population even from the hepatic functional reserve alone. BCLC intermediate stage also includes patients with multiple nodules from 4 nodules to over 10–20 bilobar tumors (table 1). Moreover, although tumor size is not clearly defined in the BCLC staging system, tumors beyond Milan criteria (single tumor >5 cm or multiple nodules ≥4) are assumed to be classified as intermediate stage. This is a very complicated situation since treatment strategy should be decided based on 3-dimensional factors such as tumor size, number and Child-Pugh score (fig. 2). An extreme ex-

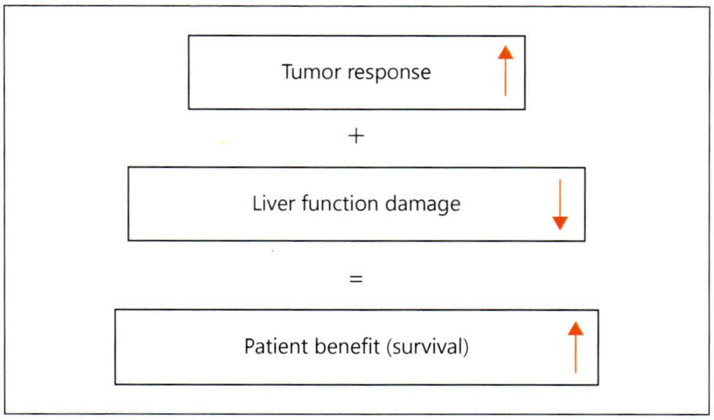

Fig. 3. Patient benefit (survival) from TACE.

ample may be that surgical resection is indicated for patients with less than 3 tumors that are slightly >3 cm in size or single tumor >5 cm, as long as they have well preserved hepatic functional reserve. A combination of preceding TACE and radiofrequency ablation (RFA) [9] can be performed in patients with ≥3 HCC nodules or a single 3–5 cm HCC. Furthermore, these large tumors may be good indications for RFA if bipolar RFA equipment is used. In addition, the aim of conventional subsegmental Lipiodol TACE (cTACE) is curative treatment, and complete response may be achieved in patients with 4–6 small tumors by superselective catheterization to a site near individual tumors, where Lipiodol and a gelatin sponge are injected, thereby inducing partial liver infarction. In other words, superselective cTACE is a highly advanced treatment technique that can be frequently used as curative treatment. However, indications for curative superselective cTACE are limited by the size and number of tumors. Therefore, it is not surprising that superselective cTACE is rarely performed in other countries, outside Japan.

Recently, the use of TACE with drug-eluting beads (DEB-TACE) that contains anti-cancer agents is becoming widespread. Specifically, DEB-TACE has been used as palliative treatment tool for mass reduction in patients who are not indicated for curative cTACE because of relatively large-sized HCCs. Because a decline in hepatic functional reserve and post-embolization syndrome are both mild after DEB-TACE as compared with cTACE, DEB-TACE is thought to be more suitable than cTACE when treating patients with a huge HCC that is >5 cm in size.

Patient benefits from TACE depend on the maximization of the tumor response as well as minimization of the liver function damage caused by TACE (fig. 3). In addition, cTACE is not only ineffective in patients with multiple lesions that have spread to both lobes, but also worsens the hepatic functional reserve of patients. These patients are supposed to benefit more from hepatic arterial infusion chemotherapy (HAIC) or sorafenib. Moreover, taking into account the limited efficacy of DEB-TACE in bilobar multinodular HCCs, it may be necessary to select HAIC as the first treatment choice for bilobar multinodular HCCs. Because preservation of liver function determines the prognosis of patients with multiple bilobar HCC nodules, treatment methods that could minimize the damage of liver function should be selected when the patient has poor hepatic liver function. Superselective cTACE is recommended even in such cases, since superselective cTACE is supposed to minimize the damage of hepatic function and maximize the tumor response.

When patients have large or many tumors and liver function reserve near 7 on the Child-Pugh scoring system, DEB-TACE or HAIC rather than cTACE is recommended to minimize the decline of hepatic function as well as to enhance treatment efficacy. In patients with a Child-Pugh score of 8–9, that is, in those with deteriorated hepatic functional reserve, we have no choice but to implement a treatment strategy that is similar to that for Child-Pugh C patients. In other words, superselective cTACE and RFA may be recommended when the number and size of tumors are limited, but in principle, BSC and possibly liver transplantation, in accordance with the extended criteria, will be indicated. For patients with favorable hepatic functional reserve and bilobar multinodular tumors, sorafenib [10, 11] is also feasible as the treatment of choice.

Subclassification of Intermediate-Stage HCC and Treatment Strategy

Because intermediate-stage HCCs encompass a heterogeneous group of patients, Bolondi et al. [12] proposed a subclassification of intermediate-stage HCCs in 2012 (table 2). This substaging system incorporates the 'beyond Milan and within up-to-7'criteria [13], a novel concept that combines the size and number of tumors, that appears to be an extremely innovative classification system. However, the substages B1, B2 and B3 are equivalent to Child-Pugh scores of 5–7, 5–6 and 7, respectively, making substaging complicated. In addition, this system basically recommends TACE as the first treatment option for B1 and B2 patients. As far as the treatment strategy (TACE) is concerned, no significant difference is observed between this substaging system and the original classification system by the BCLC staging although no

Table 2. Subgrouping and treatment indication for patients with intermediate HCC

BCLC substage	B1	B2	B3	B4
CPT score	5–6–7	5–6	7	8–9
Beyond Milan and within up-to-7	IN	OUT	OUT	ANY
ECOG (tumor-related) PS	0	0	0	0–1
PVT	NO	NO	NO	NO
1st option	TACE	TACE or TARE		BSC
Alternative	LT TACE + ablation	SOR	Research trials TACE SOR	LT

TARE = Transarterial radioembolization; SOR = sorafenib. Bolondi et al. [12].

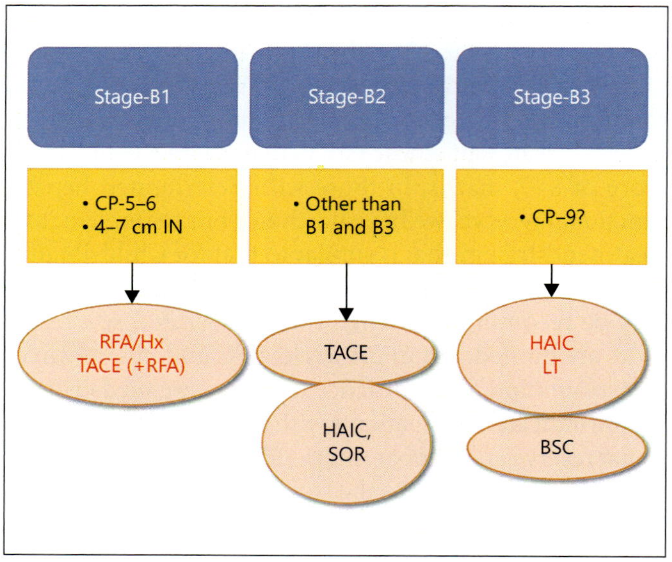

Fig. 4. Treatment guideline for BCLC-B HCC patients proposed by Japan-TAE group.

treatment option is recommended for substage B3 class and BSC is recommended for substage B4. In terms of disease prognosis, this substaging system is reportedly useful in the stratification of intermediate-stage HCC patients because prognosis worsens as substage progresses [14]. However, another report states that this subclassification is not useful [15].

Another important issue related to this substaging system is that portal vein thrombosis (PVT) is indicated as 'NO' for all B1–B4 substages. Because PVT has never been a defining factor for intermediate-stage HCC, this PVT factor should be deleted from the substaging system. Moreover, liver transplantation is recommended as an alternative treatment option for patients with Child-Pugh scores 5–7 in substage B1, but this treatment option is unrealistic because liver transplantation is not a standard of care for patients with Child-Pugh scores 5–7 in Japan. Furthermore, TACE and radioembolization are listed as the first treatment options for patients with substage B2, but radioembolization has not yet been approved in Japan. Instead, HAIC has been performed proactively in patients with bilobar multinodular HCC in Japan [16].

Apart from this subclassification, Yamakado et al. [17, 18] recommended novel subclassification criteria and treatment strategies for Japanese patients with intermediate-stage HCC in 2014 (fig. 4).

Subclassification of Intermediate-Stage HCC and Treatment Approaches: Modified Bolondi's Subclassification (Kinki Criteria)

Figure 5 shows a conceptual diagram of heterogeneity among intermediate-stage HCCs. The up-to-7 criteria are well-thought out criteria and include from single 6-cm HCC, six 1-cm nodules and nodules of in-between sizes. Therefore, this criteria uses 6 cm and 6 nodules as cutoff values, the up-to-7 criteria may also be called the 6–6 criteria.

As color-coded in green and pink represent good response subgroup to superselective cTACE and poor response subgroup to superselective cTACE, respectively (fig. 5). As color-coded in green, pink and yellow, the main treatment strategy for HCCs corresponding to Beyond Milan and within up-to-7 HCCs are curative therapy such as resection, ablation or superselective cTACE, whereas DEB-TACE is indicated for relatively large tumors. In addition, highly multiple HCCs are thought to be a good indication for HAIC or sorafenib (fig. 6).

Dig Dis 2015;33:751–758
DOI: 10.1159/000439290

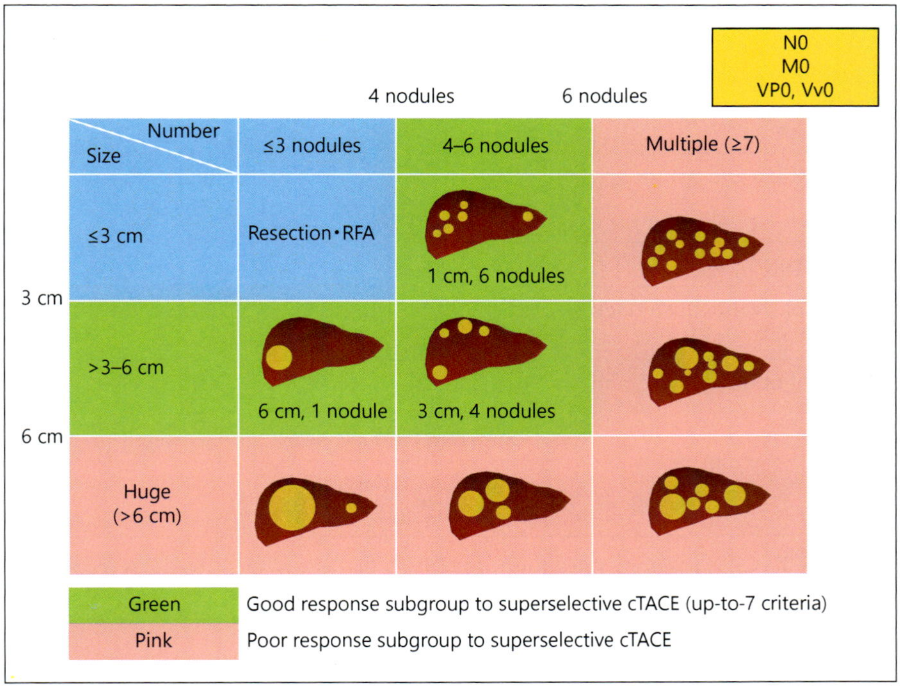

Fig. 5. Heterogeneity of intermediate stage HCC.

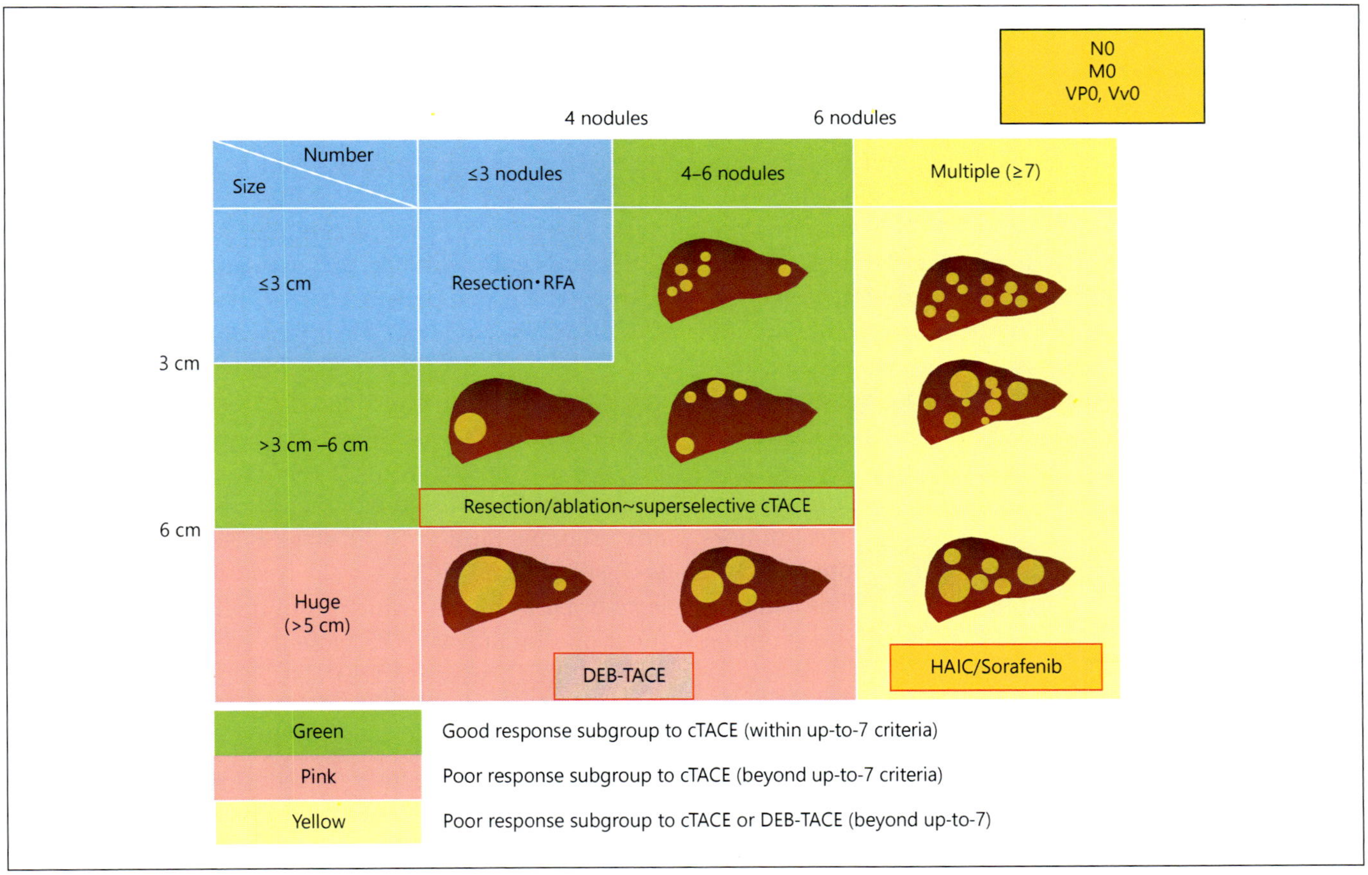

Fig. 6. Heterogeneity and treatment strategy of intermediate stage HCC (sub-stage B1, B2).

Table 3. Subclassification and treatment strategy of intermediate-stage HCC (modified Bolondi)

BCLC substage	B1	B2	B3	
Child-Pugh score	5–7	5–7	8, 9	
Beyond Milan and within up-to-7	IN	OUT	ANY	
			IN	OUT
Sub-substage			B3-a	B3-b
Concept of treatment strategy	Curative intent	Non-curative, palliative	Curative intent if within up-to-7	Palliative, no treatment
Treatment option	Resection Ablation Superselective c-TACE	DEB-TACE[1] HAIC[2] Sorafenib[3]	Transplantation Ablation Superselective cTACE	HAIC Selective DEB-TACE
Alternative	DEB-TACE (large, C-P 7) B-TACE[4]	cTACE	DEB-TACE B-TACE, HAIC	BSC

[1] DEB-TACE is recommended for huge tumors that are >6 cm. [2] HAIC is recommended for multiple tumors >6. [3] Sorafenib is recommended for patients with liver function of Child-Pugh score 5 and 6. [4] B-TACE is recommended for fewer tumors.

We have been actively utilizing a novel classification system that we developed by modifying the Bolondi's criteria [12] (table 3). In this modified Bolondi's substaging system (Kinki criteria), patients with intermediate-stage HCC are classified into 3 groups based on their Child-Pugh scores (5–7 or 8–9) and the Beyond Milan and within up-to-7 criteria (IN or OUT). Although similar to the Bolondi's substaging system to a certain extent, the Kinki criteria is simpler and easier to apply, and resection and even ablation are included as treatment options for patients with substage B1. Resection is a good treatment option for patients with well-preserved liver function corresponding to Child-Pugh score 5 and single but large tumor, while ablation may be selected for those with 4–6 small tumors. Even if tumor size is near 5 cm, ablation can be applied if preceded by TACE to make the area for ablation larger. In patients with several regional tumors, we can apply superselective cTACE to carefully treat tumors one by one with curative intent. When superselective catheterization is not applicable, DEB-TACE or Balloon-occluded TACE (B-TACE) [19] may be a choice of option (table 3; fig. 5 and 6).

In patients with substage B2 HCC that is beyond the Milan criteria and is also huge, we actively repeat DEB-TACE, which is a good treatment option for huge HCCs (fig. 6). For patients with beyond up-to-7 multiple HCCs, we select HAIC rather than DEB-TACE (fig. 6) because HAIC is effective in this group of patients. If HAIC is not effective, sorafenib may be recommended. We occasionally perform cTACE for some specific reasons but do not recommend the procedure because unselective bilobar cTACE will worsen the liver function. In addition, sorafenib may be an option for patients with numerous bilobar HCCs, who are expected to quickly become refractory to TACE. Sorafenib may be considered as the first treatment option for patients who have beyond up-to-7 bilobar multiple HCCs and are expected to easily become refractory to cTACE with worsening the liver function.

Patients with substage B3 HCCs are basically treated with a concept of palliative or no treatment similar to Child-Pugh C patients, but in those meeting the up-to-7 criteria, it is important to aim for potential cure and survival benefit, as in Child-Pugh C patients, using superselective cTACE or ablation to treat individual HCCs carefully [20]. In patients with up-to-7 HCCs, liver transplantation may be considered as extended criteria or after downstaging. Similar to substage B2 HCCs, 'within up-to-7' substage B3 HCCs may be treated with HAIC or selective DEB-TACE, which minimally decreases liver function. For substage B3 patients with beyond up-to-7 HCCs, HAIC, selective DEB-TACE or BSC are recommended (fig. 7).

We analyzed patients treated with cTACE (either superselective or unselective procedure) at our institution according to the Kinki criteria. Overall survival rates in patients with substage B1, B2 and B3 HCCs are well stratified. Because the survival curve of patients with substage B1 HCC is nearly identical to that of patients with BCLC

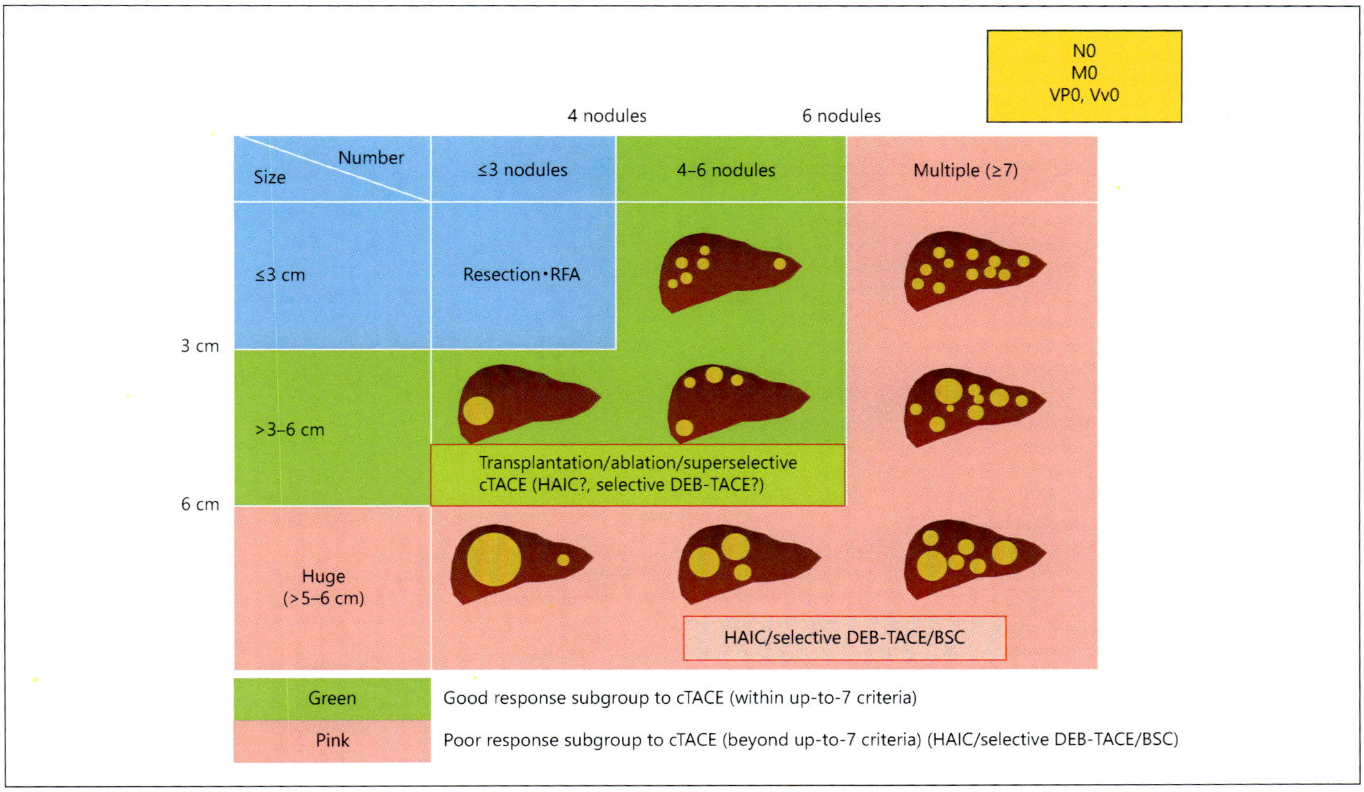

Fig. 7. Heterogeneity and treatment strategy of intermediate stage HCC (sub-stage B3). BSC = Best supportive care.

A HCC, this HCC patient subgroup should be treated with curative treatment including superselective cTACE and/or resection/ablation. As for substage B3 HCC, its survival curve overlaps with that of BCLC C, suggesting that the outcome of repeated cTACE in the patients would not be any better than that in patients with BCLC stage C HCC.

However, for substage B3 patients with tumors within up-to-7 criteria (sub-substage B3-a), superselective cTACE and ablation are recommended since these treatments have a survival benefit by minimizing the liver function damage and maximizing the treatment efficacy. Superselective/selective DEB-TACE, B-TACE, and HAIC are also indicated as alternative therapy in case of patients with sub-substage B3-a HCC.

In contrast, for patients with 'beyond up-to-7' BCLC B3 substage HCC (sub-substage B3-b), treatment options that are less toxic to liver function such as HAIC or selective DEB-TACE are indicated in accordance with the treatment results in Child-Pugh C patients [20].

However, as numbers of patients of sub-substage B3-a and B3-b are very small, it will be better to combine them as substage B3 when we analyze the survival data.

Our findings suggest that it is important to subclassify BCLC stage B HCC and establish treatment strategies based on liver function (Child-Pugh score) and tumor factors (within or beyond up-to-7).

Conclusion

In this review, heterogeneity of intermediate-stage HCCs and treatment options were discussed. Although several substaging systems have been proposed previously, we introduced here novel subclassification criteria and treatment approaches that we are currently using (Kinki criteria) by modifying Bolondi's subclassification. Further study is needed to retrospectively investigate how well our system stratifies intermediate-stage HCCs and to prospectively determine the validity of this modified Bolondi's subclassification, Kinki criteria.

Disclosure Statement

Authors declare there is no conflict of interest.

References

1 Bruix J, Sherman M; American Association for the Study of Liver Diseases: Management of hepatocellular carcinoma: an update. Hepatology 2011;53:1020–1022.

2 European Association for the Study of the Liver; European Organisation for Research and Treatment of Cancer: EASL-EORTC clinical practice guidelines: management of hepatocellular carcinoma. J Hepatol 2012;56: 908–943.

3 Kokudo N, Hasegawa K, Akahane M, Igaki H, Izumi N, Ichida T, Uemoto S, Kaneko S, Kawasaki S, Ku Y, Kudo M, Kubo S, Takayama T, Tateishi R, Fukuda T, Matsui O, Matsuyama Y, Murakami T, Arii S, Okazaki M, Makuuchi M: Evidence-based clinical practice guidelines for hepatocellular carcinoma: the Japan society of hepatology 2013 update (3rd JSH-HCC guidelines). Hepatol Res 2015; 45.

4 Kudo M, Matsui O, Izumi N, Iijima H, Kadoya M, Imai Y, Okusaka T, Miyayama S, Tsuchiya K, Ueshima K, Hiraoka A, Ikeda M, Ogasawara S, Yamashita T, Minami T, Yamakado K; Liver Cancer Study Group of Japan: JSH consensus-based clinical practice guidelines for the management of hepatocellular carcinoma: 2014 update by the liver cancer study group of Japan. Liver Cancer 2014; 3:458–468.

5 Kudo M: Clinical practice guidelines for hepatocellular carcinoma differ between Japan, United States, and Europe. Liver Cancer 2015; 4:85–95.

6 Omata M, Lesmana LA, Tateishi R, Chen PJ, Lin SM, Yoshida H, Kudo M, Lee JM, Choi BI, Poon RT, Shiina S, Cheng AL, Jia JD, Obi S, Han KH, Jafri W, Chow P, Lim SG, Chawla YK, Budihusodo U, Gani RA, Lesmana CR, Putranto TA, Liaw YF, Sarin SK: Asian Pacific association for the study of the liver consensus recommendations on hepatocellular carcinoma. Hepatol Int 2010;4:439–474.

7 Minami Y, Yagyu Y, Murakami T, Kudo M: Tracking navigation imaging of transcatheter arterial chemoembolization for hepatocellular carcinoma using three-dimensional conebeam CT angiography. Liver Cancer 2014;3: 53–61.

8 Raoul JL, Gilabert M, Piana G: How to define transarterial chemoembolization failure or refractoriness: a European perspective. Liver Cancer 2014;3:119–124.

9 Lin SM: Local ablation for hepatocellular carcinoma in Taiwan. Liver Cancer 2013;2:73–83.

10 Peck-Radosavljevic M: Drug therapy for advanced-stage liver cancer. Liver Cancer 2014; 3:125–131.

11 Kudo M: Biomarkers and personalized sorafenib therapy. Liver Cancer 2014;3:399–404.

12 Bolondi L, Burroughs A, Dufour JF, Galle PR, Mazzaferro V, Piscaglia F, Raoul JL, Sangro B: Heterogeneity of patients with intermediate (BCLC B) hepatocellular carcinoma: proposal for a subclassification to facilitate treatment decisions. Semin Liver Dis 2012;32:348–359.

13 Mazzaferro V, Llovet JM, Miceli R, Bhoori S, Schiavo M, Mariani L, Camerini T, Roayaie S, Schwartz ME, Grazi GL, Adam R, Neuhaus P, Salizzoni M, Bruix J, Forner A, De Carlis L, Cillo U, Burroughs AK, Troisi R, Rossi M, Gerunda GE, Lerut J, Belghiti J, Boin I, Gugenheim J, Rochling F, Van Hoek B, Majno P; Metroticket Investigator Study Group: Predicting survival after liver transplantation in patients with hepatocellular carcinoma beyond the Milan criteria: a retrospective, exploratory analysis. Lancet Oncol 2009;10:35–43.

14 Scaffaro LA, Stella SF, Alvares-Da-Silva MR, Kruel CD: Survival rates according to Barcelona clinic liver cancer sub-staging system after transarterial embolization for intermediate hepatocellular carcinoma. World J Hepatol 2015;7:628–632.

15 Weinmann A, Koch S, Sprinzl M, Kloeckner R, Schulze-Bergkamen H, Düber C, Lang H, Otto G, Wörns MA, Galle PR: Survival analysis of proposed BCLC-B subgroups in hepatocellular carcinoma patients. Liver Int 2015;35: 591–600.

16 Kudo M: Treatment of advanced hepatocellular carcinoma with emphasis on hepatic arterial infusion chemotherapy and molecular targeted therapy. Liver Cancer 2012;1: 62–70.

17 Yamakado K, Miyayama S, Hirota S, Mizunuma K, Nakamura K, Inaba Y, Maeda H, Matsuo K, Nishida N, Aramaki T, Anai H, Koura S, Oikawa S, Watanabe K, Yasumoto T, Furuichi K, Yamaguchi M: Subgrouping of intermediate-stage (BCLC stage B) hepatocellular carcinoma based on tumor number and size and Child-Pugh grade correlated with prognosis after transarterial chemoembolization. Jpn J Radiol 2014;32:260–265.

18 Yamakado K, Miyayama S, Hirota S, Mizunuma K, Nakamura K, Inaba Y, Yamamoto S, Matsuo K, Nishida N, Aramaki T, Anai H, Kora S, Oikawa S, Watanabe K, Yasumoto T, Furuichi K, Yamaguchi M: Prognosis of patients with intermediate-stage hepatocellular carcinomas based on the Child-Pugh score: subclassifying the intermediate stage (Barcelona clinic liver cancer stage B). Jpn J Radiol 2014;32:644–649.

19 Irie T, Kuramochi M, Takahashi N: Dense accumulation of lipiodol emulsion in hepatocellular carcinoma nodule during selective balloon-occluded transarterial chemoembolization: measurement of balloon-occluded arterial stump pressure. Cardiovasc Intervent Radiol 2013;36:706–713.

20 Kudo M, Osaki Y, Matsunaga T, Kasugai H, Oka H, Seki T: Hepatocellular carcinoma in Child-Pugh C cirrhosis: prognostic factors and survival benefit of nontransplant treatments. Dig Dis 2013;31:490–498.

Review Article

Digestive Diseases

Dig Dis 2015;33:759–764
DOI: 10.1159/000439100

Cone-Beam CT Angiography for Hepatocellular Carcinoma: Current Status

Yasunori Minami[a] Takamichi Murakami[b] Masayuki Kitano[a]
Toshiharu Sakurai[a] Naoshi Nishida[a] Masatoshi Kudo[a]

Departments of [a]Gastroenterology and Hepatology and [b]Radiology, Kinki University School of Medicine, Osaka-Sayama, Osaka, Japan

Key Words

Cone-beam CT angiography · Hepatocellular carcinoma · Maximum intensity projection · Transcatheter arterial chemoembolization · Volume rendering

Abstract

Cone-beam CT (CBCT) is generated during a rotational sweep of the C-arm around the patient, and can be a valuable imaging technique, providing in situ cross-sectional imaging. It is easy to evaluate the morphologic characteristics of hepatic arteries from multiple views with the use of various reconstruction techniques, such as maximum intensity projection (MIP) and volume rendering. CBCT angiography is capable of providing more information than the standard 2-dimensional angiography in visualizing hepatocellular carcinomas (HCCs) and targeting tumors though precise microcatheter placement in close proximity to HCCs. It can also be useful in evaluating treatment success at the time of the procedure. It is anticipated that CBCT could reduce radiation exposure, the overall procedure time and contrast material use because it allows immediate feedback for an efficient angiographic procedure. Therefore, CBCT angiography is an exciting technology with the potential to significantly impact the practice of interventional radiology. The purpose of this article is to provide a review of the principles, clinical applications and technique of CBCT angiography for HCC treatment.

Introduction

Transcatheter arterial chemoembolization (TACE) is the first-line therapy recommended for patients with intermediate hepatocellular carcinoma (HCC) [1–8]. Selective catheterization of a target artery is a prerequisite for achieving effective TACE in HCC patients. However, it is often difficult to determine the relationship between multiple overlapping vessels from 2-dimensional (2D) angiographic images [9–11]. Furthermore, small vessels may be obscured when they are adjacent to large areas of opacification. When complex vascular structures are being imaged, it may be necessary to make multiple acquisitions at various angles to provide adequate visualization. However, multiple acquisitions result in increased radiation exposure to the patient and repeated injections of contrast material. To minimize these angiography risks, it is crucial to provide the operator with a 3-dimensional (3D) representation of the patient's liver along with its vasculature and lesions.

Over the past decade, interventional radiology (IVR)-CT angiography and cone-beam CT (CBCT) angiography have been introduced as 3D angiography systems. The IVR-CT angiography system consists of angiography and a multidetector row CT (MDCT) unit, and is conducted with the patient on the same bed without risking dislodgment of the catheter [12, 13]. IVR-CT angiography offers high-resolution images of the vascular anatomy or the shape and volume of the vascular territories [14–16]. However, these systems are only found in a lim-

KARGER 125

E-Mail karger@karger.com
www.karger.com/ddi

0257–2753/15/0336–0759$39.50/0

Masatoshi Kudo, MD, PhD
Department of Gastroenterology and Hepatology
Kinki University School of Medicine
377-2 Ohno-Higashi, Osaka-Sayama, Osaka 589-8511 (Japan)
E-Mail m-kudo@med.kindai.ac.jp

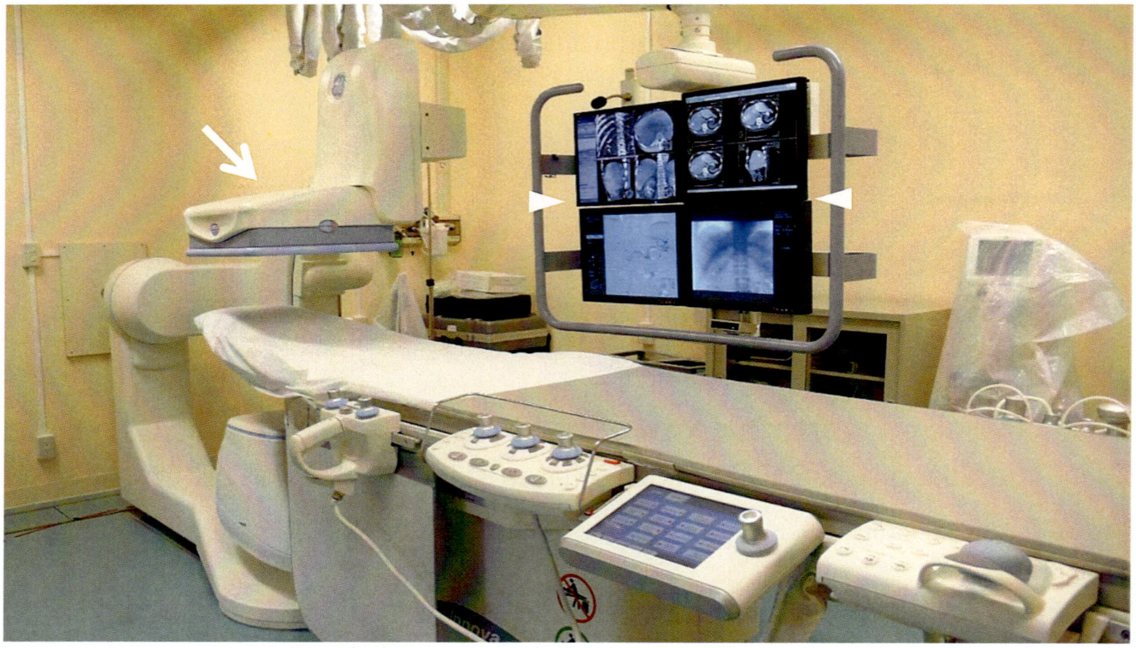

Fig. 1. C-arm-mounted FPD CBCT system. The C-arm equipped with a FPD (arrow) is aligned with the table. The large monitor (arrow heads) can show patient monitoring information and different imaging inputs, including live fluoroscopy, 2D angiography and the results of the embolization planning and guidance software overlaid on live fluoroscopy images.

ited number of hospitals because they are rather expensive and require a great deal of space. On the other hand, the CBCT system consists of a C-arm gantry, an X-ray tube and a flat-panel detector (FPD), and can offer great flexibility in orienting the detector around the patient. CBCT is able to provide the benefit of space and time savings while offering good 3D angiography.

This article summarizes the principles, clinical applications and technique of CBCT angiography for HCC treatment.

CBCT Angiography

System

CBCT mounted on a C-arm was originally performed using an image intensifier system. However, image intensifier systems and charged couple devices suffer from limited spatial resolution. The FPD-based system replaced the image intensifier system during the 1990s. The development of FPD has provided significantly high resolution, high detector quantum efficiency, high frame rate, high dynamic range, small image lag and excellent linearity in comparison with image intensifier detectors [17]. Recent FPDs cover a planar region of 19 × 25 cm and up to 40 × 40 cm for a reconstructed volume of 25 × 25 × 19 cm to 40 × 40 × 40 cm at a high spatial resolution on the order of 150 × 150 μm^2 pixel size. Furthermore, CBCT allows for lower radiation and intravenous contrast doses by FPD. CBCT imaging is based on a projection acquisition, whereby a cone-shaped X-ray beam and FPD are mounted on a C-arm gantry (fig. 1). This configuration provides projection radiography, fluoroscopy, digital subtraction angiography (DSA) and volumetric CT capabilities in a single patient setup, within the interventional suite. Such capabilities allow the operator to perform intraprocedural volumetric imaging without the need for patient transportation to a CT unit.

The FPD C-arm CBCT data are generated during a rotational sweep of C-arm around the patient. X-ray projection images of the object are acquired in multiple angular directions, following a circular path covering an angular range of at least 200°. The target area is positioned at the center of rotation and CBCT volumes are then obtained by integrating information from the 2D high-resolution projection images.

Generally, the contrast-to-noise ratio of CBCT images is 1.5–2 times lower when compared with that of MDCT, primarily due to less-advanced anti-scatter radiation technology [18, 19]. On the other hand, due to the finer detector pitch, its spatial resolution is superior. This combina-

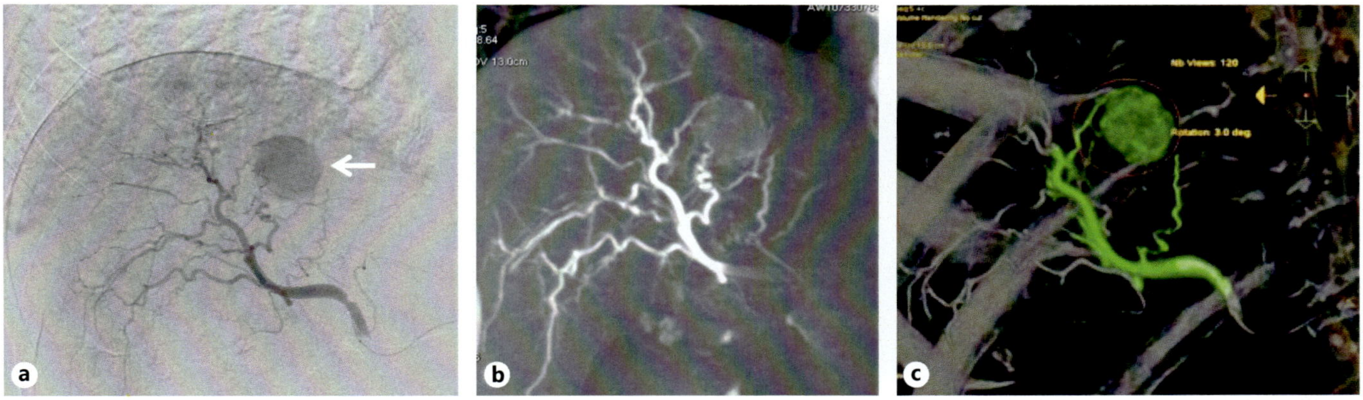

Fig. 2. A 74-year-old man with an HCC of 3.0 cm diameter. **a** 2D angiography shows HCC as an enhanced lesion (arrow) complicated with right anterior hepatic arteries. **b** Thin-slab MIP image (slab thickness = 20 mm) permits visualization of small branch vessels, and also shows the HCC to be more complicated, with right anterior hepatic arteries. **c** Two green vessels indicate the tumor feeding arteries from the right anterior hepatic artery to HCC by the automatic tracking navigation imaging with volume rendering.

tion of high spatial resolution and intra-arterial administration of iodinated contrast material compensates for the lower contrast resolution and provides a high-quality tumor depiction along with detailed vascular anatomy.

Imaging Technique Options

CBCT has been shown to be a valuable imaging technique, providing in situ cross-sectional imaging of CT-like quality [20]. The reconstructed 3D DSA images show only the enhanced vascular lumina, and data are stored. Therefore, it is easy to evaluate the morphologic characteristics of the hepatic arteries from multiple views with the use of various reconstruction techniques, such as maximum intensity projection (MIP) and volume rendering [21].

MIP

MIP is a specific type of rendering in which the brightest voxel is projected into the 3D image. MIP image allows the differentiation between enhanced vascular structures and non-vascular structures, because the result is a projection of the highest density. CT angiographic applications for which the use of MIP is advantageous include the creation of a vascular map for display by a referring physician and easy visualization of small intraparenchymal branches in an enhancing organ, such as the liver or kidney [22]. In practice, MIP is usually performed interactively with a sliding slab, enabling the radiologist to adjust the window, select the optimal orientation to display each artery and modify the slab thickness. This sliding thin-slab MIP technique has been found to increase sensitivity in the detection of lung nodules and arteriovenous malformations [23, 24].

Volume Rendering

Volume rendering can better depict soft tissues and 3D relationships because volume rendering can display a set of data in its entirety. This property allows volume-rendered CT angiograms to provide vessel 'depth' and to display multiple overlapping vessels, more effectively excluding the surrounding structures [21, 25]. In addition, volume rendering allows for a color display, which often improves the visualization of complex anatomies and 3D relationships. Small vessels are more accurately depicted with volume rendering, and MIP may not be. Recently, the medical imaging community has embraced volume rendering for a wide variety of 3D imaging applications including this navigation imaging on CBCT.

Tracking Navigation Imaging

The tracking navigation software is an advanced vascular 3D clinical analysis tool using data from CBCT angiography [26]. There are 2 software programs (Flight Plan for Liver, GE Healthcare, Chalfont St Gilles, England, or EmboGuide, Philips Healthcare, Best, The Netherlands), and these 3D navigation tools can automatically depict all vessels in the vicinity of the target as being feeding arteries (fig. 2). Tracking navigation imaging can highlight all vessels (from the tip of the microcatheter to the tumor) that appeared to feed the tumor by coming into close geometric proximity with the region of interest. Moreover, virtual '3D roadmap' imaging can superimpose the live fluoroscopic images with 3D reconstruction in the GE system. The 3D roadmap is automatically adjusted in real time for all changes in C-arm angu-

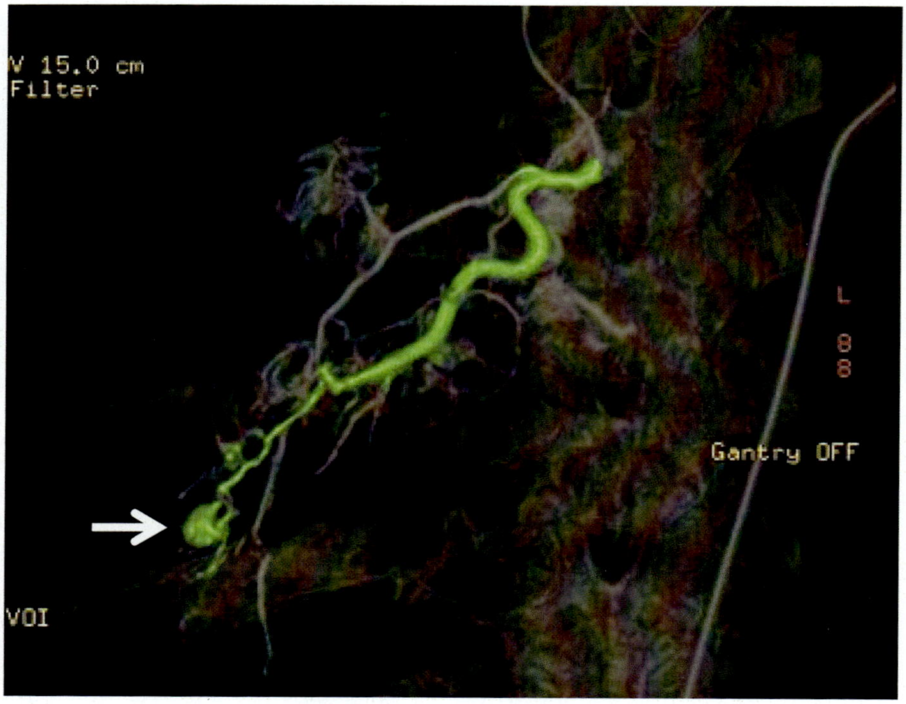

Fig. 3. A 77-year-old man with hemoptysis. Volume rendering shows right brachial artery, and green vessel depicts the active extravasation of contrast material. Tracking navigation imaging can be available for other organs except the liver.

lations, field of view and table positions. The operator can move the C-arm into an optimal position that best facilitates catheterization and minimizes vessel overlap and foreshortening, without losing the matching between live fluoroscopy and the angiographic roadmap.

Clinical Outcomes

Special information about the feeding vessels of HCC is helpful for successful catheterization and sufficient TACE. Kakeda et al. [27] reported that CBCT provided additional useful information in 42 of the 52 lesions (81%) for therapeutic decision making or TACE compared with DSA. Miyayama et al. [28] showed that the sensitivity of CBCT in the detection of the tumor-feeding artery is superior to that of non-selective DSA (81 vs. 38%, $p < 0.01$). The availability of CBCT volumetric information can be used to achieve comprehensive visualization of the hepatic arterial anatomy and tumor feeding arteries and to determine the degree of selectivity of drug delivery to the targeted tumors, thus reducing the risk of non-target embolization and potential complications.

Recent developments in software programming have enabled automatic identification of the feeding vessels on 3D angiography. The TACE procedure can be carried out completely in patients with complicated vessels of the liver by color coding the feeding vessels. Miyayama et al. [28] reported on automatic feeder vessel detection software with a true-positive ratio of 88% in identifying the tumor feeding artery. Iwazawa et al. [29] also showed that the sensitivity in detecting tumor feeders was 87.7%. Therefore, automatic computed analysis software is able to achieve greater than 90% sensitivity in tumor feeding artery detection of hypervascular HCC lesions, which is 29–50% higher than visual identification on a nonselective DSA study [26, 30–33]. Automated software may also be used to detect parasitic feeding artery from other than the proper hepatic artery and the cystic artery and select the optimal microcatheter position for drug delivery to avoid non-target embolization [34] (fig. 3).

Unenhanced CBCT after conventional TACE is known as Lip-CBCT, and Lip-CBCT is a technique used to assess the lipiodol deposition in the tumor after conventional TACE. Lip-CBCT imaging provides immediate feedback to the operator with lipiodol conspicuity equivalent to unenhanced MDCT and is predictive of tumor response when compared with 1-month follow-up multiphasic MDCT or contrast-enhanced MRI [31, 35, 36]. The use of Lip-CBCT helps to achieve complete iodized oil filling of HCCs, and therefore improves therapeutic effects by optimizing the embolization end point [36]. Intraprocedural Lip-CBCT depicts HCC with 100% sensitivity compared with preprocedural diagnostic imaging [31]. Poor iodized oil accumulation on Lip-CBCT may be an unfavorable predictor in HCC patients treated with conventional TACE.

Conclusion

C-arm CBCT is an exciting technology with the potential to significantly impact the practice of IVR. CBCT angiography is capable of providing more information than the standard 2D angiography in visualizing HCCs and targeting tumors though precise microcatheter placement in close proximity to HCCs. It can also be useful in evaluating treatment success at the time of the procedure. CBCT is based on immediate feedback to the angiographic procedure. Therefore, CBCT can inspire greater confidence and should be useful for TACE in HCC patients with complicated feeding arteries.

Disclosure Statement

The authors declare that no conflict of interest exists.

References

1 Nakamura H, Hashimoto T, Oi H, Sawada S: Transcatheter oily chemoembolization of hepatocellular carcinoma. Radiology 1989;170 (3 pt 1):783–786.

2 Matsui O, Kadoya M, Yoshikawa J, Gabata T, Arai K, Demachi H, Miyayama S, Takashima T, Unoura M, Kogayashi K: Small hepatocellular carcinoma: treatment with subsegmental transcatheter arterial embolization. Radiology 1993;188:79–83.

3 Takayasu K, Arii S, Ikai I, Omata M, Okita K, Ichida T, Matsuyama Y, Nakanuma Y, Kojiro M, Makuuchi M, Yamaoka Y; Liver Cancer Study Group of Japan: Prospective cohort study of transarterial chemoembolization for unresectable hepatocellular carcinoma in 8,510 patients. Gastroenterology 2006;131:461–469.

4 Llovet JM, Real MI, Montaña X, Planas R, Coll S, Aponte J, Ayuso C, Sala M, Muchart J, Solà R, Rodés J, Bruix J; Barcelona Liver Cancer Group: Arterial embolisation or chemoembolisation versus symptomatic treatment in patients with unresectable hepatocellular carcinoma: a randomised controlled trial. Lancet 2002;359:1734–1739.

5 Sergio A, Cristofori C, Cardin R, Pivetta G, Ragazzi R, Baldan A, Girardi L, Cillo U, Burra P, Giacomin A, Farinati F: Transcatheter arterial chemoembolization (TACE) in hepatocellular carcinoma (HCC): the role of angiogenesis and invasiveness. Am J Gastroenterol 2008;103:914–921.

6 Ueda T, Murata S, Yasui D, Mine T, Kumita S: Comparison of the antitumor efficacy of transcatheter arterial chemoembolization with a miriplatin-iodized oil suspension and a cisplatin-iodized oil suspension for hepatocellular carcinoma. Hepatol Res 2013;43:1071–1077.

7 Lencioni R: Chemoembolization in patients with hepatocellular carcinoma. Liver Cancer 2012;1:41–50.

8 Kudo M, Matsui O, Izumi N, Iijima H, Kadoya M, Imai Y, Okusaka T, Miyayama S, Tsuchiya K, Ueshima K, Hiraoka A, Ikeda M, Ogasawara S, Yamashita T, Minami T, Yamakado K; Liver Cancer Study Group of Japan: JSH Consensus-based clinical practice guidelines for the management of hepatocellular carcinoma: 2014 update by the Liver Cancer Study Group of Japan. Liver Cancer 2014;3:458–468.

9 Lewandowski RJ, Geschwind JF, Liapi E, Salem R: Transcatheter intraarterial therapies: rationale and overview. Radiology 2011;259: 641–657.

10 Lencioni R, Crocetti L: Local-regional treatment of hepatocellular carcinoma. Radiology 2012;262:43–58.

11 Bouvier A, Ozenne V, Aubé C, Boursier J, Vullierme MP, Thouveny F, Farges O, Vilgrain V: Transarterial chemoembolisation: effect of selectivity on tolerance, tumour response and survival. Eur Radiol 2011;21:1719–1726.

12 Takayasu K, Muramatsu Y, Maeda T, Iwata R, Furukawa H, Muramatsu Y, Moriyama N, Okusaka T, Okada S, Ueno H: Targeted transarterial oily chemoembolization for small foci of hepatocellular carcinoma using a unified helical CT and angiography system: analysis of factors affecting local recurrence and survival rates. AJR Am J Roentgenol 2001; 176:681–688.

13 Toyoda H, Kumada T, Sone Y: Impact of a unified CT angiography system on outcome of patients with hepatocellular carcinoma. AJR Am J Roentgenol 2009;192:766–774.

14 Nelson RC, Chezmar JL, Sugarbaker PH, Bernardino ME: Hepatic tumors: comparison of CT during arterial portography, delayed CT, and MR imaging for preoperative evaluation. Radiology 1989;172:27–34.

15 Kanematsu M, Hoshi H, Imaeda T, Murakami T, Inaba Y, Yokoyama R, Nakamura H: Detection and characterization of hepatic tumors: value of combined helical CT hepatic arteriography and CT during arterial portography. AJR Am J Roentgenol 1997;168:1193–1198.

16 Murakami T, Oi H, Hori M, Kim T, Takahashi S, Tomoda K, Narumi Y, Nakamura H: Helical CT during arterial portography and hepatic arteriography for detecting hypervascular hepatocellular carcinoma. AJR Am J Roentgenol 1997;169:131–135.

17 Ning R, Chen B, Yu R, Conover D, Tang X, Ning Y: Flat panel detector-based cone-beam volume CT angiography imaging: system evaluation. IEEE Trans Med Imaging 2000;19:949–963.

18 Paul J, Jacobi V, Farhang M, Bazrafshan B, Vogl TJ, Mbalisike EC: Radiation dose and image quality of X-ray volume imaging systems: cone-beam computed tomography, digital subtraction angiography and digital fluoroscopy. Eur Radiol 2013;23:1582–1593.

19 Gonzalez-Guindalini FD, Ferreira Botelho MP, Töre HG, Ahn RW, Gordon LI, Yaghmai V: MDCT of chest, abdomen, and pelvis using attenuation-based automated tube voltage selection in combination with iterative reconstruction: an intrapatient study of radiation dose and image quality. AJR Am J Roentgenol 2013;201:1075–1082.

20 Orth RC, Wallace MJ, Kuo MD; Technology Assessment Committee of the Society of Interventional Radiology: C-arm cone-beam CT: general principles and technical considerations for use in interventional radiology. J Vasc Interv Radiol 2008;19:814–820.

21 Fishman EK, Ney DR, Heath DG, Corl FM, Horton KM, Johnson PT: Volume rendering versus maximum intensity projection in CT angiography: what works best, when, and why. Radiographics 2006;26:905–922.

22 Soyer P, Heath D, Bluemke DA, Choti MA, Kuhlman JE, Reichle R, Fishman EK: Three-dimensional helical CT of intrahepatic venous structures: comparison of three rendering techniques. J Comput Assist Tomogr 1996;20:122–127.

23 Ertl-Wagner BB, Bruening R, Blume J, Hoffmann RT, Mueller-Schunk S, Snyder B, Reiser MF: Relative value of sliding-thin-slab multiplanar reformations and sliding-thin-slab maximum intensity projections as reformatting techniques in multisection CT angiography of the cervicocranial vessels. AJNR Am J Neuroradiol 2006;27:107–113.

Dig Dis 2015;33:759–764
DOI: 10.1159/000439100

24 Kawel N, Seifert B, Luetolf M, Boehm T: Effect of slab thickness on the CT detection of pulmonary nodules: use of sliding thin-slab maximum intensity projection and volume rendering. AJR Am J Roentgenol 2009;192:1324–1329.
25 Calhoun PS, Kuszyk BS, Heath DG, Carley JC, Fishman EK: Three-dimensional volume rendering of spiral CT data: theory and method. Radiographics 1999;19:745–764.
26 Deschamps F, Solomon SB, Thornton RH, Rao P, Hakime A, Kuoch V, de Baere T: Computed analysis of three-dimensional cone-beam computed tomography angiography for determination of tumor-feeding vessels during chemoembolization of liver tumor: a pilot study. Cardiovasc Intervent Radiol 2010;33:1235–1242.
27 Kakeda S, Korogi Y, Ohnari N, Moriya J, Oda N, Nishino K, Miyamoto W: Usefulness of cone-beam volume CT with flat panel detectors in conjunction with catheter angiography for transcatheter arterial embolization. J Vasc Interv Radiol 2007;18:1508–1516.
28 Miyayama S, Yamashiro M, Hashimoto M, Hashimoto N, Ikuno M, Okumura K, Yoshida M, Matsui O: Identification of small hepatocellular carcinoma and tumor-feeding branches with cone-beam CT guidance technology during transcatheter arterial chemoembolization. J Vasc Interv Radiol 2013;24:501–508.
29 Iwazawa J, Ohue S, Hashimoto N, Muramoto O, Mitani T: Clinical utility and limitations of tumor-feeder detection software for liver cancer embolization. Eur J Radiol 2013;82:1665–1671.
30 Loffroy R, Lin M, Rao P, Bhagat N, Noordhoek N, Radaelli A, Blijd J, Geschwind JF: Comparing the detectability of hepatocellular carcinoma by C-arm dual-phase cone-beam computed tomography during hepatic arteriography with conventional contrast-enhanced magnetic resonance imaging. Cardiovasc Intervent Radiol 2012;35:97–104.
31 Miyayama S, Yamashiro M, Okuda M, Yoshie Y, Sugimori N, Igarashi S, Nakashima Y, Matsui O: Usefulness of cone-beam computed tomography during ultraselective transcatheter arterial chemoembolization for small hepatocellular carcinomas that cannot be demonstrated on angiography. Cardiovasc Intervent Radiol 2009;32:255–264.
32 Higashihara H, Osuga K, Onishi H, Nakamoto A, Tsuboyama T, Maeda N, Hori M, Kim T, Tomiyama N: Diagnostic accuracy of C-arm CT during selective transcatheter angiography for hepatocellular carcinoma: comparison with intravenous contrast-enhanced, biphasic, dynamic MDCT. Eur Radiol 2012;22:872–879.
33 Minami Y, Yagyu Y, Murakami T, Kudo M: Tracking navigation imaging of transcatheter arterial chemoembolization for hepatocellular carcinoma using three-dimensional cone-beam CT angiography. Liver Cancer 2014;3:53–61.
34 Wang X, Shah RP, Maybody M, Brown KT, Getrajdman GI, Stevenson C, Petre EN, Solomon SB: Cystic artery localization with a three-dimensional angiography vessel tracking system compared with conventional two-dimensional angiography. J Vasc Interv Radiol 2011;22:1414–1419.
35 Chen R, Geschwind JF, Wang Z, Tacher V, Lin M: Quantitative assessment of lipiodol deposition after chemoembolization: comparison between cone-beam CT and multidetector CT. J Vasc Interv Radiol 2013;24:1837–1844.
36 Monsky WL, Kim I, Loh S, Li CS, Greasby TA, Deutsch LS, Badawi RD: Semiautomated segmentation for volumetric analysis of intratumoral ethiodol uptake and subsequent tumor necrosis after chemoembolization. AJR Am J Roentgenol 2010;195:1220–1230.

Review Article

Digestive Diseases

Dig Dis 2015;33:765–770
DOI: 10.1159/000439101

General Rules for the Clinical and Pathological Study of Primary Liver Cancer, Nationwide Follow-Up Survey and Clinical Practice Guidelines: The Outstanding Achievements of the Liver Cancer Study Group of Japan

Masatoshi Kudo Masayuki Kitano Toshiharu Sakurai Naoshi Nishida

Department of Gastroenterology and Hepatology, Kinki University School of Medicine, Osaka-Sayama, Osaka, Japan

Key Words

Primary liver cancer · Hepatocellular carcinoma · Practice guideline · General rules · Locoregional therapy · Response evaluation criteria in cancer of the liver

Abstract

This review outlines the significance of establishing general rules, a nationwide follow-up survey, and clinical practice guidelines for liver cancer in Japan. The general rules are an essential part of hepatocellular carcinoma (HCC) treatment, enabling a 'common language' to be used in daily clinical practice and for the nationwide follow-up survey. The Japanese General Rules for the Clinical and Pathological Study of Primary Liver Cancer, which provide detailed descriptions of HCC, are excellent and are unique to Japan. Items in the General Rules for the Clinical and Pathological Study of Primary Liver Cancer are used substantially in another important project, the Nationwide Follow-Up Survey of Primary Liver Cancer, which has been rigorously undertaken with great effort by the Liver Cancer Study Group of Japan biannually since 1969. Both evidence-based and consensus-based treatment algorithms for HCC are used to complement each other in clinical practice in Japan.

Introduction

As for other cancers, general rules and clinical practice guidelines have been developed for hepatocellular carcinoma (HCC). Historically, the general rules for HCC have been published by the Liver Cancer Study Group of Japan (LCSGJ), under the title 'General Rules for the Clinical and Pathological Study of Primary Liver Cancer'. After the publication of the first edition on June 20, 1983, subsequent editions were published in 1987 (2nd edition), 1992 (3rd edition), 2001 (4th edition) and 2008 (5th edition), followed by a revision of the current fifth edition on July 7, 2009 [1, 2]. The sixth edition is scheduled for publication in 2015. While the general rules for other cancers have been compiled primarily by the respective large medical societies, the general rules for primary liver cancer were published by the LCSGJ.

In terms of the clinical practice guidelines for HCC, the Clinical Practice Guidelines Committee for Liver Cancer (Chairman, Dr. Masatoshi Makuuchi), sponsored by the Ministry of Health, Labour and Welfare, played a central role in establishing the first edition of the Evidence-based Clinical Practice Guidelines for HCC in 2005. The committee consisted mainly of executive council members of the LCSGJ. Thereafter, the Japan Society

KARGER 125

© 2015 S. Karger AG, Basel
0257–2753/15/0336–0765$39.50/0

E-Mail karger@karger.com
www.karger.com/ddi

Masatoshi Kudo, MD, PhD
Department of Gastroenterology and Hepatology
Kinki University School of Medicine, 377-2 Ohno-Higashi
Osaka-Sayama, Osaka 589-8511 (Japan)
E-Mail m-kudo@med.kindai.ac.jp

of Hepatology (JSH) sponsored the publication of the second edition of the guidelines in 2009 and the latest edition in 2013 [3]. JSH also published the first and second editions of the Clinical Practice Manual for HCC, 'Management of Hepatocellular Carcinoma in Japan: Consensus-Based Clinical Practice Manual' in 2007 and the revised version in 2010, respectively [4, 5]. The third edition was published in 2015 [6, 7]. This manual is useful as it incorporates recommendations with a high level of evidence that are presented in the aforementioned Evidence-based Clinical Practice Guidelines for HCC [8–10], while also explaining diagnoses and treatments relevant to routine clinical settings that are in line with expert opinion and consensus.

General Rules for the Clinical and Pathological Study of Primary Liver Cancer

The first edition of General Rules for the Clinical and Pathological Study of Primary Liver Cancer was published to provide physicians specializing in liver cancer with specific terminology and abbreviations for noting the macroscopic findings of HCC, tumor stage, pathological findings, important terminology and the accompanying cirrhosis state and also for enabling discussions using 'common language'. Every time a subsequent edition was published, the TNM classification system became unique to Japan, and owing to advances in pathological studies, the definition of pathological early well-differentiated HCC [11] was clearly stated already in the third edition published in 1992. Moreover, Japan has adopted the liver damage to reflect degree of liver functional reserve, instead of the Child-Pugh classification, which is a global standard. This unique approach has arisen because the indocyanine green retention test is frequently performed before surgical resection in Japan. In that sense, liver damage is more of an HCC-oriented liver functional reserve classification than Child-Pugh classification, where the latter was originally developed to predict the prognosis of cirrhotic patients [12, 13].

With the publication of the General Rules for the Clinical and Pathological Study of HCC and Intrahepatic Cholangiocarcinoma in Japanese and English, unique advances have been made. The TNM classification of HCC and intrahepatic cholangiocarcinoma is easy to remember and judge because the staging of T1–T4 tumors involves only 3 criteria: <2 or ≥2 cm, the presence or absence of vascular invasion and single or multiple tumors (table 1). This innovative staging system is again unique to Japan and differentiates itself from the TNM classification system used worldwide that was developed by the Union for International Cancer Control (UICC) and American Joint Committee on Cancer. A study that used the TNM classification systems proposed by the LCSGJ and the UICC to examine Japanese patients showed that the former system allowed for more accurate stratification [14]. This also demonstrates that Japan's General Rules for the Clinical and Pathological Study of Primary Liver Cancer have developed in a unique way.

Table 1. Definitions of the TNM stage by the LCSGJ

Stage I	T1 (fulfilling 3 T factors) N0 M0
Stage II	T2 (fulfilling 2 T factors) N0 M0
Stage III	T3 (fulfilling 1 T factors) N0 M0
Stage IV-A	T4 (fulfilling 0 T factors) N0 M0
Stage IV-B	Any T N0–1 M1

T factor: (1) single, (2) <2 cm and (3) no vascular involvement.

These General Rules for the Clinical and Pathological Study of Primary Liver Cancer are important not only in providing a 'common language' for hepatologists, surgeons, pathologists and radiologists involved in the treatment of liver cancer to use, but also in unifying the description of survey items in the Nationwide Follow-Up Survey of Primary Liver Cancer, which is another large project run by the LCSGJ since its establishment in 1967. This huge database is an extremely important asset that is not available in any other country. Because HCC was treated only by surgical resection [15–17] in the 1970s before locoregional therapy [18–22] was developed in the 1980s, the general rules describe surgery-related items and the macroscopic and histopathological findings of surgical specimens in immense detail. In contrast, descriptions of locoregional therapies, such as ablation [21] and transcatheter arterial chemoembolization (TACE) [13, 23, 24], were relatively scarce up until the fourth edition, which was published in 2001. However, due to the rapid progress of these therapies for HCC, there was an urgent need to introduce terminology or descriptions about locoregional therapy and to establish detailed response evaluation criteria for treatment. These changes were made in the 2009 revision of the fifth edition. The outcome of treatment for HCC has conventionally been evaluated using the Response Evaluation Criteria for the Solid Tumors (RECIST), which was developed to assess the treatment response of other solid tumors. RECIST is not suitable though for evaluat-

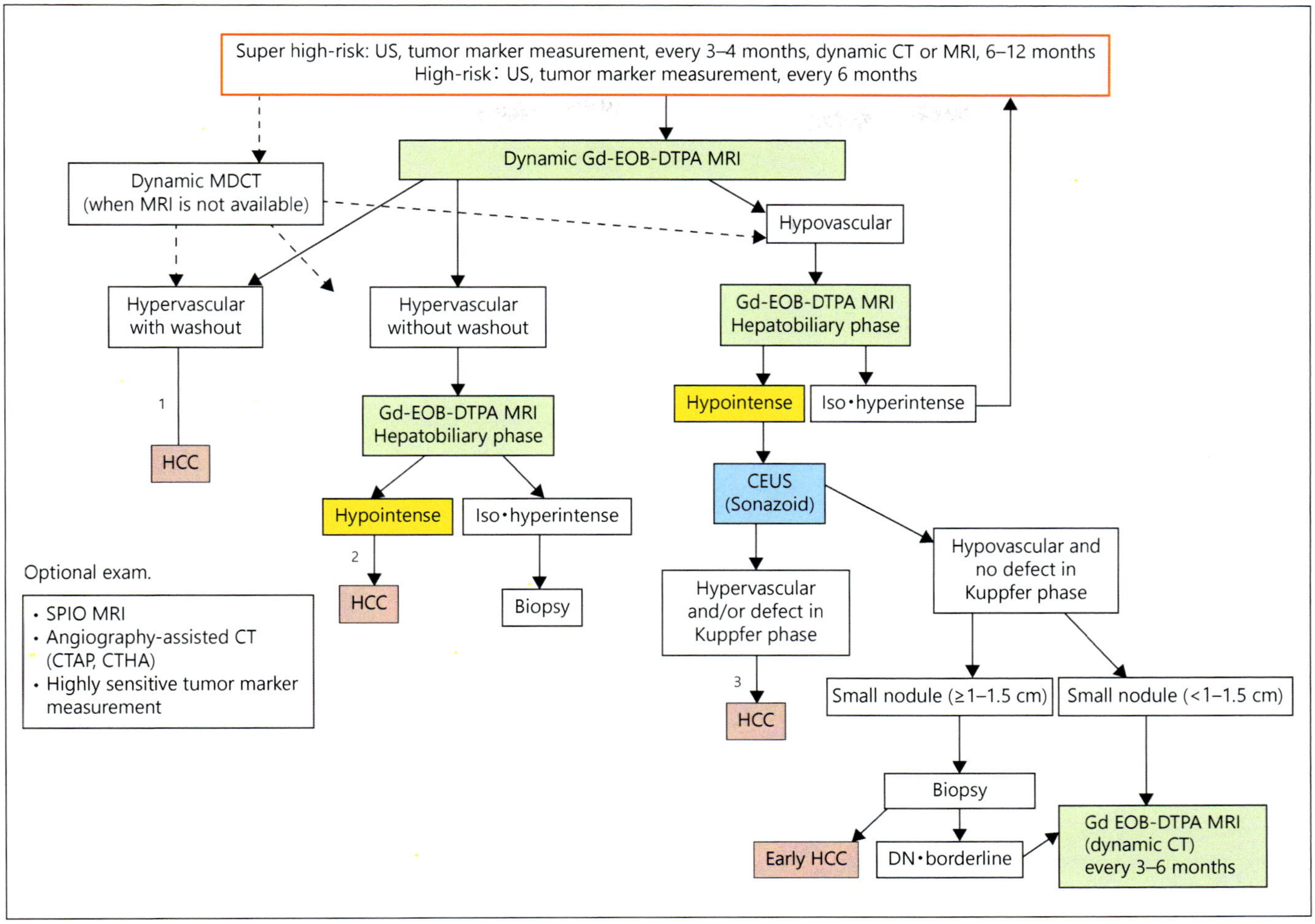

Fig. 1. Surveillance and diagnostic algorithm of HCC (proposed by LCSGJ 2014). [1] Cavernous hemangioma may show hypointensity on equilibrium (transitional) phase of dynamic Gd-EOB-DTPA MRI (pseudo-washout). It should be excluded by other sequences of MRI and/or other imaging modalities. [2] Cavernous hemangioma usually shows hypointensity on hepatobiliary phase of Gd-EOB-DTPA MRI. It should be excluded by other sequences of MRI and/or other imaging modalities. [3] Biopsy may be considered for confirmation.

ing the treatment response of HCC. Therefore, the LCSGJ has developed unique criteria to evaluate the direct treatment effects by locoregional therapies such as ablation or TACE. However, following recent advances in systemic chemotherapy using the molecular targeted agent, sorafenib, the fifth edition was revised to include the response evaluation of systemic therapy and was reissued under the title 'Response Evaluation Criteria in Cancer of the Liver' (RECICL) [25] in order to apply the criteria and to evaluate the outcome of systemic chemotherapy.

The forthcoming sixth edition of the general rules in 2015 will include the revision of the TNM classification system for intrahepatic cholangiocarcinoma, descriptions of lymph node metastasis and HCC rupture and more sophisticated revised response evaluation criteria, namely, RECICL version 1.1 [26]. These revisions will also improve the descriptions used in the follow-up survey, thus making all the revision efforts worthwhile.

Clinical Practice Guidelines

The essential elements of the Evidence-Based Clinical Practice Guidelines for Liver Cancer are the surveillance, diagnostic and treatment algorithms for HCC. The guidelines also cover prevention, diagnosis, surveillance, surgery, ablation therapy, TACE, systemic chemotherapy [27, 28], radiation therapy [29, 30], post-treatment follow-up, prevention of recurrence after curative treatment

Dig Dis 2015;33:765–770
DOI: 10.1159/000439101

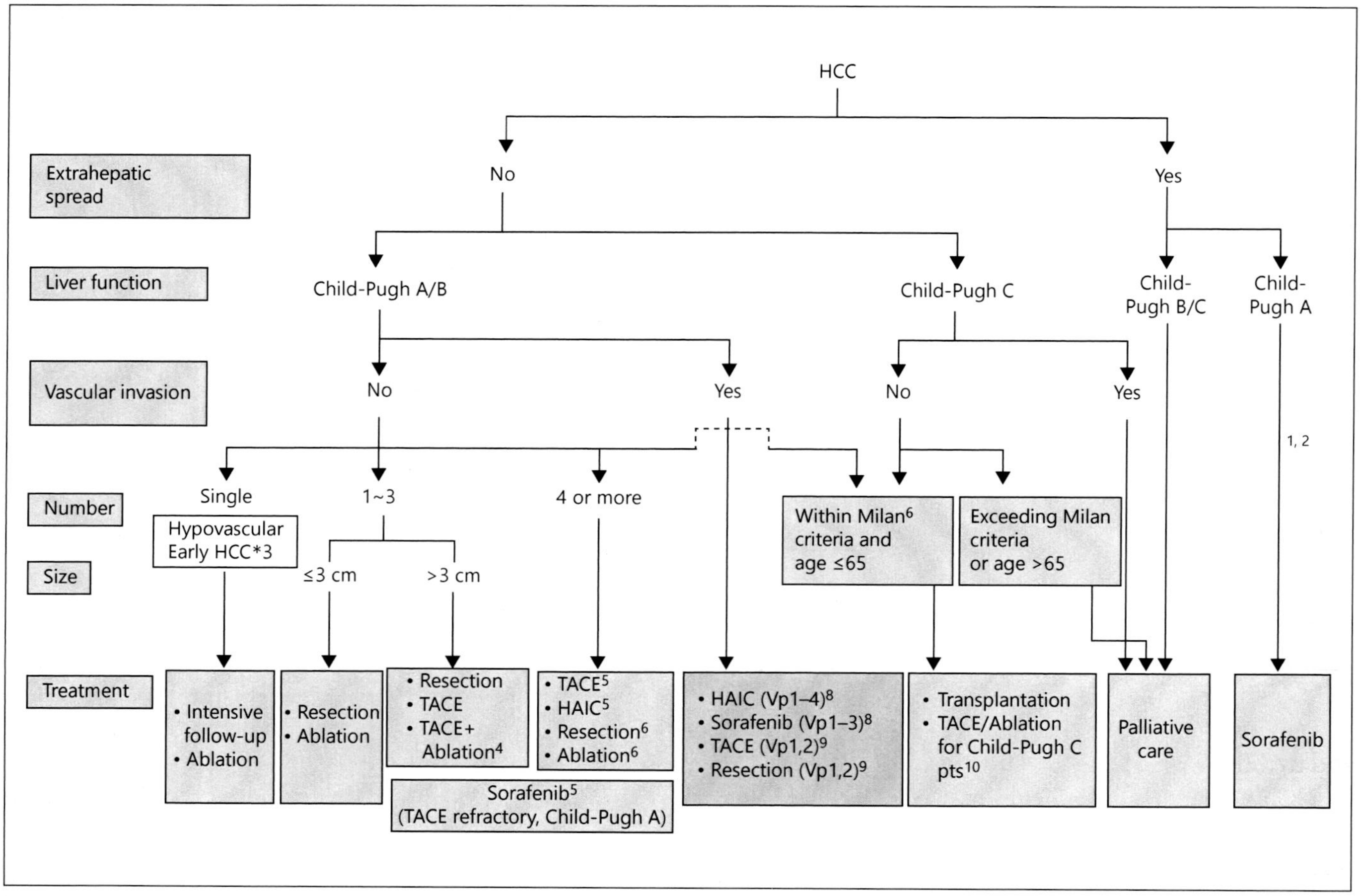

Fig. 2. JSH-LCSGJ consensus-based treatment algorithm for HCC revised in 2014. [1] Treatment should be performed as if extrahepatic spead is negative, when extrahepatic spread is not regarded as a prognostic factor. [2] Sorafenib is the first choice of treatment in this setting as a standard of care. [3] Intensive follow-up observation is recommended for hypovascular nodules by the Japanese Evidence-Based Clinical Practice Guidelines. However, local ablation therapy is frequently performed in the following cases: (1) when the nodule is diagnosed pathologically as early HCC; (2) when the nodules show decreased uptake on hepatocyte phase Gd-EOB-MRI; (3) when the nodules show decreased portal flow by CTAP or (4) decreased uptake is shown on Kupffer phase of Sonazoid enhanced US, since these nodules are known to frequently progress to the typical hypervascular HCC. [4] Even for HCC nodules exceeding 3 cm in diameter, combination therapy of TACE and ablation is frequently performed when resection is not indicated. [5] Transcathetherarterial chemoembolization (TACE) is the first choice of treatment in this setting. Hepatic arterial infusion chemotherapy (HAIC) using an implanted port is also recommended for TACE refractory patients . The regimen for this treatment is usually low-dose FP (5FU + CDDP) or intraarterial 5FU infusion combined with systemic interferon therapy. Sorafenib is also a treatment of choice for TACE refractory patients with Child Pugh A liver function. [6] Resection is sometimes performed even when numbers of nodules are over 4. Furthermore, ablation is sometimes performed in combination with TACE. [7] Milan criteria: Tumor size <3 cm and tumor numbers <3; or solitary tumor <5 cm. Even when liver function is good (Child-Pugh A/B), transplantation is sometimes considered for frequently recurring HCC patients. [8] Sorafenib and HAIC are recommended for HCC patients with Vp1,2 (minor portal vein invasion), Vp3 (portal invasion at the 1st portal branch). Sorafenib is not recommended for HCC patients with Vp4 (portal invasion at the main portal branch), whereas HAIC is recommended for such patients with tumor thrombus in the main portal branch. [9] Resection and TACE is frequently performed when portal invasion is minimum such as Vp1(portal invasion at the 3rd or more peripheral portal branch) or Vp2 (portal invasion at the 2nd portal branch). [10] Local ablation therapy or subsegmental TACE is performed even for Child-Pugh C patients when transplantation is not indicated when there is no hepatic encephalopathy, no uncontrollable ascites, and a low bilirubin level (<3.0 mg/dl). Although it is as a well accepted treatment in the routine clinical setting, there is no evidence of its survival benefit in Child-Pugh C patients. A prospective study is necessary to clarify this issue. Even in Child-Pugh A/B patients, transplantation is sometimes performed for relatively younger patients with frequently or early recurring HCC after curative treatments.

Table 2. Definition of TACE failure/refractoriness (LCSGJ)

1	Intrahepatic lesion (i) Two or more consecutive insufficient responses within the treated tumors (viable lesion >50%) even after changing the chemotherapeutic agents and/or re-analysis of feeding artery can be seen by response evaluation CT/MRI after the 1–3 months following adequately performed selective TACE (ii) Two or more consecutive progression in the liver (tumor numbers even increase as compared to the tumor numbers before the previous TACE procedure) even after changing the chemotherapeutic agents and/or re-analysis of feeding artery can be seen by response evaluation CT/MRI after the 1–3 months following adequately performed selective TACE
2	Tumor marker Continuous elevation of tumor markers right after TACE even though transient minor reduction is observed
3	Appearance of vascular invasion
4	Appearance of extrahepatic spread

and treatment for recurrence. These issues are introduced in a 'Clinical Questions' format, in which questions routinely asked in daily clinical practice are answered based on facts with a high level of evidence that are reported in scientific articles selected during an extensive review of the literature. Evidence levels and recommended grades are listed to assist the diagnosis and treatment of HCC in daily clinical practice. The surveillance and diagnostic algorithm, the most important part of the clinical practice guidelines, recommends regular ultrasound and tumor marker screening using 3 markers (AFP, AFP-L3 and PIVKA-II) [31–33] or annual-to-semiannual CT or MRI depending on whether the patients are categorized as very high-risk or high-risk patients. The treatment algorithm presents treatment strategies that are in line with the severity of liver damage and the number and size of tumors [8, 9]. The 2013 edition states that the Child-Pugh classification can be used when non-surgical therapy is applied [3, 10].

But, it should be noted that, since the consensus-based surveillance and diagnostic algorithm is relatively complex, it is scheduled to be simplified considerably in the 2015 edition (fig. 1) [7]. This was the results of consensus meeting at the 50th Annual Meeting of LCSGJ (Congress President: Prof. Masatoshi Kudo). In addition, the proposed treatment algorithm provides extremely useful guidance for daily clinical practice because it contains a list of practical treatment strategies that are being performed in accordance with current treatment policies developed based on expert opinion and consensus (fig. 2). The criteria for TACE failure/refractoriness were also included in the third edition of the guidelines (table 2) [34].

It was revealed at the 48th LCSGJ Congress (Congress President, Prof. Osamu Matsui, Kanazawa University) [35] that over 90% of physicians specializing in liver cancer who diagnose and treat liver cancer refer to the JSH's Evidence-based Clinical Practice Guidelines for HCC or Consensus-based Clinical Practice Guidelines for HCC. This indicates how well these guidelines complement each other and assist in optimizing diagnosis and treatment of liver cancer in Japan.

Conclusion

This review outlines the significance of establishing general rules, a nationwide follow-up survey and clinical practice guidelines for liver cancer in Japan. The general rules are an essential part of HCC treatment, enabling a 'common language' to be used in daily clinical practice and for the nationwide follow-up survey. The Japanese General Rules for the Clinical and Pathological Study of Primary Liver Cancer [2], which provide detailed descriptions of HCC, are excellent and are unique to Japan. Items in the General Rules for the Clinical and Pathological Study of Primary Liver Cancer are used substantially in another important project, the Nationwide Follow-Up Survey of Primary Liver Cancer which has been rigorously undertaken with great effort by the LCSGJ biannually since 1969.

Both the evidence-based and consensus-based treatment algorithms for HCC are used to complement each other in clinical practice in Japan. The most important point going forward is that prospective clinical trials are needed to accumulate solid evidence for the recommendations proposed in the consensus-based treatment algorithm, which are not included in the evidence-based clinical practice guidelines because of the lack of such evidence. In fact, clinical trials are now looking for evidence, and include the SURF trial (UMIN No. UMIN000001795), SILIUS trial (NCT Trial No. 01214343), TACTICS trial (NCT Trial No. 01217034) and DELICATE trial. Their results are eagerly awaited.

Disclosure Statement

The authors declare that they have no conflict of interest.

References

1 The Liver Cancer Study Group of Japan: The General Rules for the Clinical and Pathological Study of Primary Liver Cancer, ed 5, Rivised Version. Tokyo, Kanehara, 2009.

2 Liver Cancer Study Group of Japan: General Rules for the Clinical and Pathological Study of Primary Liver Cancer, ed 3. Tokyo, Kanehara & Co., Ltd., 2010.

3 Japan Society of Hepatology: Evidence-Based Clinical Practice Guidelines for Hepatocellular Carcinoma. Tokyo, Kanehara & Co., 2013.

4 Japan Society of Hepatology: Management of Hepatocellular Carcinoma in Japan: Consensus-Based Clinical Practice Manual, ed 2. Tokyo, Igaku-Shoin, 2010.

5 Kudo M, Izumi N, Kokudo N, Matsui O, Sakamoto M, Nakashima O, Kojiro M, Makuuchi M: Management of hepatocellular carcinoma in Japan: consensus-based clinical practice guidelines proposed by the Japan society of hepatology (JSH) 2010 updated version. Dig Dis 2011;29:339–364.

6 Chow PK: Intra-arterial radiotherapy for advanced HCC with vascular invasion. Liver Cancer 2014;3:213.

7 Kudo M, Matsui O, Izumi N, Iijima H, Kadoya M, Imai Y, Okusaka T, Miyayama S, Tsuchiya K, Ueshima K, Hiraoka A, Ikeda M, Ogasawara S, Yamashita T, Minami T, Yamakado K; Liver Cancer Study Group of Japan: JSH consensus-based clinical practice guidelines for the management of hepatocellular carcinoma: 2014 update by the Liver Cancer Study Group of Japan. Liver Cancer 2014;3:458–468.

8 Kokudo N, Makuuchi M: Evidence-based clinical practice guidelines for hepatocellular carcinoma in Japan: the J-HCC guidelines. J Gastroenterol 2009;44(suppl 19):119–121.

9 Makuuchi M, Kokudo N, Arii S, Igaki H, Ikai I, Kaneko S, Kawasaki S, Kudo M, Matsuyama Y, Ohtomo K, Okazaki M, Omata M, Takayama T, Takayasu K, Tateishi R: Surveillance algorithm and diagnostic algorithm for hepatocellular carcinoma. Hepatol Res 2010;40: 1–144.

10 Kokudo N, Hasegawa K, Akahane M, Igaki H, Izumi N, Ichida T, Uemoto S, Kaneko S, Kawasaki S, Ku Y, Kudo M, Kubo S, Takayama T, Tateishi R, Fukuda T, Matsui O, Matsuyama Y, Murakami T, Arii S, Okazaki M, Makuuchi M: Evidence-based clinical practice guidelines for hepatocellular carcinoma: the Japan society of hepatology 2013 update (3rd JSH-HCC guidelines). Hepatol Res 2015; 45.

11 Kudo M: Early hepatocellular carcinoma: definition and diagnosis. Liver Cancer 2013;2: 69–72.

12 Clinical practice guidelines for hepatocellular carcinoma differ between Japan, United States, and Europe. Liver Cancer 2015;4:85–95.

13 Kudo M: Surveillance, diagnosis, treatment, and outcome of liver cancer in Japan. Liver Cancer 2015;4:39–50.

14 Makuuchi M, Belghiti J, Belli G, Fan ST, Lau JW, Ringe B, Strasberg SM, Vauthey JN, Yamaoka Y, Yamasaki S: IHPBA concordant classification of primary liver cancer: working group report. J Hepatobiliary Pancreat Surg 2003;10:26–30.

15 Mise Y, Sakamoto Y, Ishizawa T, Kaneko J, Aoki T, Hasegawa K, Sugawara Y, Kokudo N: A worldwide survey of the current daily practice in liver surgery. Liver Cancer 2013;2:55–66.

16 Shindoh J, Kaseb A, Vauthey JN: Surgical strategy for liver cancers in the era of effective chemotherapy. Liver Cancer 2013;2:47–54.

17 Kubo S, Takemura S, Sakata C, Urata Y, Uenishi T: Adjuvant therapy after curative resection for hepatocellular carcinoma associated with hepatitis virus. Liver Cancer 2013;2:40–46.

18 Minami Y, Yagyu Y, Murakami T, Kudo M: Tracking navigation imaging of transcatheter arterial chemoembolization for hepatocellular carcinoma using three-dimensional conebeam CT angiography. Liver Cancer 2014;3: 53–61.

19 Khajornjiraphan N, Thu NA, Chow PK: Yttrium-90 microspheres: a review of its emerging clinical indications. Liver Cancer 2015;4: 6–15.

20 Kudo M: Locoregional therapy for hepatocellular carcinoma. Liver Cancer 2015;4:163–164.

21 Lin SM: Local ablation for hepatocellular carcinoma in Taiwan. Liver Cancer 2013;2:73–83.

22 Teng W, Liu KW, Lin CC, Jeng WJ, Chen WT, Sheen IS, Lin CY, Lin SM: Insufficient ablative margin determined by early computed tomography may predict the recurrence of hepatocellular carcinoma after radiofrequency ablation. Liver Cancer 2015;4:26–38.

23 Raoul JL, Gilabert M, Piana G: How to define transarterial chemoembolization failure or refractoriness: a European perspective. Liver Cancer 2014;3:119–124.

24 Edeline J, Gilabert M, Garin E, Boucher E, Raoul JL: Yttrium-90 microsphere radioembolization for hepatocellular carcinoma. Liver Cancer 2015;4:16–25.

25 Kudo M, Kubo S, Takayasu K, Sakamoto M, Tanaka M, Ikai I, Furuse J, Nakamura K, Makuuchi M: Response evaluation criteria in cancer of the liver (RECICL) proposed by the Liver Cancer Study Group of Japan (2009 revised version). Hepatol Res 2010;40:686–692.

26 Kudo M, Ueshima K, Kubo S, Sakamoto M, Tanaka M, Ikai I, Furuse J, Murakami T, Kadoya M, Kokudo N: Response evaluation criteria in cancer of the liver (RECICL) (2015 revised version). Hepatol Res 2015, Epub ahead of print.

27 Peck-Radosavljevic M: Drug therapy for advanced-stage liver cancer. Liver Cancer 2014; 3:125–131.

28 Siegel AB, El-Khoueiry AB, Finn RS, Guthrie KA, Goyal A, Venook AP, Blanke CD, Verna EC, Dove L, Emond J, Kato T, Samstein B, Busuttil R, Remotti H, Coffey A, Brown RS Jr: Phase I trial of sorafenib following liver transplantation in patients with high-risk hepatocellular carcinoma. Liver Cancer 2015;4:115–125.

29 Lee DS, Seong J: Radiotherapeutic options for hepatocellular carcinoma with portal vein tumor thrombosis. Liver Cancer 2014;3:18–30.

30 Choi C, Choi GH, Kim TH, Tanaka M, Meng MB, Seong J: Multimodality management for Barcelona clinic liver cancer stage C hepatocellular carcinoma. Liver Cancer 2014;3:405–416.

31 Kudo M: Alpha-fetoprotein-L3: useful or useless for hepatocellular carcinoma? Liver Cancer 2013;2:151–152.

32 Toyoda H, Kumada T, Tada T, Sone Y, Kaneoka Y, Maeda A: Tumor markers for hepatocellular carcinoma: simple and significant predictors of outcome in patients with HCC. Liver Cancer 2015;4:126–136.

33 Song P, Gao J, Inagaki Y, Kokudo N, Hasegawa K, Sugawara Y, Tang W: Biomarkers: evaluation of screening for and early diagnosis of hepatocellular carcinoma in Japan and china. Liver Cancer 2013;2:31–39.

34 Kudo M, Matsui O, Izumi N, Kadoya M, Okusaka T, Miyayama S, Yamakado K, Tsuchiya K, Ueshima K, Hiraoka A, Ikeda M, Ogasawara S, Yamashita T, Minami T: Transarterial chemoembolization failure/refractoriness: JSH-LCSGJ criteria 2014 update. Oncology 2014;87(suppl 1):22–31.

35 Kudo M, Matsui O, Sakamoto M, Kitao A, Kim T, Ariizumi S, Ichikawa T, Kobayashi S, Imai Y, Izumi N, Fujinaga Y, Arii S: Role of gadolinium-ethoxybenzyl-diethylenetriamine pentaacetic acid-enhanced magnetic resonance imaging in the management of hepatocellular carcinoma: consensus at the symposium of the 48th annual meeting of the Liver Cancer Study Group of Japan. Oncology 2013;84(suppl 1):21–27.

Review Article

Digestive Diseases

Dig Dis 2015;33:771–779
DOI: 10.1159/000439102

Molecular Mechanism and Prediction of Sorafenib Chemoresistance in Human Hepatocellular Carcinoma

Naoshi Nishida   Masayuki Kitano   Toshiharu Sakurai   Masatoshi Kudo

Department of Gastroenterology and Hepatology, Kinki University School of Medicine, Osaka-Sayama, Osaka, Japan

Key Words

Hepatocellular carcinoma · Chemoresistance · Sorafenib · Signaling pathway · MicroRNA · Apoptosis · Immunity · Cancer stem cell · Epithelial-mesenchymal transition

Abstract

Hepatocellular carcinoma (HCC) is the second leading cause of cancer death worldwide, and prognosis remains unsatisfactory when the disease is diagnosed at an advanced stage. Many molecular targeted agents are being developed for the treatment of advanced HCC; however, the only promising drug to have been developed is sorafenib, which acts as a multi-kinase inhibitor. Unfortunately, a subgroup of HCC is resistant to sorafenib, and the majority of these HCC patients show disease progression even after an initial satisfactory response. To date, a number of studies have examined the underlying mechanisms involved in the response to sorafenib, and trials have been performed to overcome the acquisition of drug resistance. The anti-tumor activity of sorafenib is largely attributed to the blockade of the signals from growth factors, such as vascular endothelial growth factor receptor and platelet-derived growth factor receptor, and the downstream RAF/mitogen-activated protein/extracellular signal-regulated kinase (ERK) kinase (MEK)/ERK cascade. The activation of an escape pathway from RAF/MEK/ERK possibly results in chemoresistance. In addition, there are several features of HCCs indicating sorafenib resistance, such as epithelial-mesenchymal transition and positive stem cell markers. Here, we review the recent reports and focus on the mechanism and prediction of chemoresistance to sorafenib in HCC.

Introduction

Hepatocellular carcinoma (HCC) is the second leading cause of cancer death [1], and prognosis of advanced HCC, such as vascular invasion and extrahepatic metastasis, is unsatisfactory. To date, sorafenib is the only molecular targeted agent that has improved the time to progression and overall survival in advanced HCC cases [2]. According to the previous reports, only a small number of patients show a regression of tumor after the initiation of sorafenib treatment, suggesting that the main action of the drug is the induction of a dormant state of tumor [3–5]. Nevertheless, a considerable number of HCCs are refractory to sorafenib, and such patients show unfavorable prognosis with reduced survival as their tumor progresses. In this review, we focus on the molecular mechanisms of acquiring chemoresistance to sorafenib and also discuss the molecular profile that predicts the effect of this promising molecular targeted agent.

Naoshi Nishida, MD, PhD
Department of Gastroenterology and Hepatology
Kinki University School of Medicine, 377-2 Ohno-Higashi
Osaka-Sayama, Osaka 589-8511 (Japan)
E-Mail naoshi@med.kindai.ac.jp

Disruption of TGF-β Pathway and Epithelial-Mesenchymal Transition Phenotype

Activation of TGF-β pathway is known to be associated with the acquisition of epithelial-mesenchymal transition (EMT) and chemoresistance in cancer cells. Recently, it was reported that HCC cell lines with an EMT-like phenotype and high expression of the stem cell marker, CD44, are refractory to sorafenib-induced cell death [6]. Therefore, it is plausible that EMT and expression of the stem cell markers induced by activation of the TGF-β pathway could be a predictor of unfavorable response of sorafenib in HCC. Another report has shown that the activation of TGF-β induces the expression of stress-responsive long non-coding RNA (lncRNA), which could impair chemotherapy-induced cell death and induce cells positive for the stem cell marker, CD133 [7]. Interestingly, sorafenib also induces stress-responsive lncRNA expression in treated cells [7], suggesting that acquisition of chemoresistance to sorafenib may involve the disruption of TGF-β, a stress-responsive lncRNA.

Alteration of PI3K/Akt Pathway

Akt signaling regulates several fundamental cellular functions including survival, proliferation, metabolism and migration. Activation of the phosphoinositide 3-kinase/protein kinase K (PI3K/Akt) pathway and alteration of its regulator has been observed in many types of cancer including HCC, and constitutive activation of Akt could induce chemoresistance in cancer cells. In addition, activation of the PI3K/Akt pathway is involved in the acquisition of stem cell-like properties and EMT phenotype in HCC through the induction of microRNA (miR)-216a/217 [8]. It was shown that expression of miR-216a/217 in tumor tissues was associated with disease-free survival, and cell lines expressing these miRs displayed an EMT phenotype. MiR-216a/217 targets phosphatase and tensin homolog (PTEN) and mothers against decapentaplegic homolog 7 (SMAD7), and inhibition of PTEN and SMAD7 with miR-216a/217 leads to the activation of PI3K/Akt and TGF-β pathways, which should result in an acquired resistance to sorafenib [8].

Alteration of RAF/MEK/ERK Pathway

The RAF/mitogen-activated protein/extracellular signal-regulated kinase (ERK) kinase (MEK)/ERK cascade is activated by growth signals and frequently dysregulated in many types of cancer. Originally, it was reported that sorafenib inhibited tumor cell proliferation and survival by blocking the canonical pathway of RAF/MEK/ERK [9]. Therefore, detecting alteration of the molecules involved in this pathway could be a promising approach for predicting sorafenib resistance. However, somatic mutations of the genes in this pathway are not frequent, even in recent analyses performed using next-generation sequencers [10].

We have reported that amplification of the *cyclin D1 (CCND1)* gene is associated with aggressive tumor behavior [11]. Focal amplification of fibroblast growth factor (FGF)-CCND1 locus, containing *FGF3, FGF4, FGF19, Janus kinase-3 (JAK3)* and *CCND1*, is reportedly observed in HCCs that show complete response to sorafenib treatment, whereas amplification is not detected in patients showing disease progression [12, 13]. It was also elucidated that cancer cell lines with FGF3/FGF4- or FGF receptor 2-amplification display hypersensitivity to sorafenib [12]. Therefore, constitutive activation of the FGF signal could predict response to sorafenib. In addition to the aberrant signaling of growth factors and receptors, inactivation of Ras effectors that act as tumor suppressors, such as Ras-association domain family 1A (RASSF1A) and NORE1A (RASSF5), could also induce activation of the RAF/MEK/ERK pathway. We have reported that transcription of RASSF family genes is frequently silenced through DNA methylation in HCC tissues [14–17]. A further report suggested that NORE1A could sensitize cancer cells to sorafenib-induced apoptosis [18]. As it has also been shown that epigenetic silencing of NORE1A is observed in HCC [18, 19], and methylation of NORE1A could represent a predictor of sorafenib resistance.

On the contrary, several miRs exert a tumor suppressive function by targeting growth factor receptors. For example, miR-224 and miR-122 inhibit tumor growth and sensitize HCC cells to sorafenib through the down-regulation of platelet-derived growth factor receptor and insulin-like growth factor 1 receptor, which could lead to increased progression-free survival of HCC [20, 21].

Escape Pathway of Classical RAF/MEK/ERK Cascade

Several reports have suggested that sorafenib resistance should, at least partially, be attributed to activation of the escape pathway of canonical RAF/MEK/ERK pathway. It is reported that aberrant activation of epidermal growth factor receptor (EGFR)/human epidermal growth factor receptor 3 (HER3) is observed in cells that have acquired sorafenib resistance [22]. In this case, constitutive activation of ERK as well as Akt should take place and result in chemoresistance to sorafenib. Therefore, activation of the PI3K/Akt pathway could be a marker of sorafenib resistance as described above, and combined

Dig Dis 2015;33:771–779
DOI: 10.1159/000439102

treatment with gefitinib and sorafenib could regulate both ERK and Akt and improve cellular chemosensitivity [22]. Xia et al. [8] also showed that activation of the PI3K/Akt pathway leads to the induction of EMT, cancer stem cell-like properties and sorafenib resistance through the suppression of PTEN by miR-216a/217. However, as discussed above, one of the effects of the Ras regulator, NORE1A, is to induce sorafenib-induced apoptosis, which requires the activation of the mammalian sterile 20-like kinase-1/Akt pathway [18]. Therefore, the role of the Akt pathway in the acquisition of sorafenib resistance remains controversial. It is possible that cross talk with other signaling pathway results in the controversial results regarding the role of Akt in sorafenib resistance.

We also reported that activation of c-jun N-terminal kinase (JNK) was significantly higher in HCC patients who were non-responsive than that in patients who responded to sorafenib [23]. The activation of JNK was correlated with the increased expression of the stem cell marker CD133. Moreover, inhibition of JNK reduced the growth of CD133-positive HCC cells, suggesting that JNK activation could induce chemoresistance to sorafenib via induction of CD133-positive cells, and that JNK inhibitors may represent a candidate drug for the treatment of sorafenib-resistant HCCs.

Recently, Rudalska et al. [24] identified molecules associated with sorafenib resistance in liver cancer using RNA interference screening of the genes located in an amplified region of human HCC. In particular, they showed that the *Mapk14* gene is involved in chemoresistance to sorafenib. The product of the *Mapk14* gene, p38α, is one of the mitogen-activated protein kinases (MAPKs) involved in the alternative downstream proliferation signal. Interestingly, the authors also showed crosstalk between p38α and downstream, a target of RAF. Therefore, inhibition of RAF by sorafenib may give rise to activation of p38α, which leads to the acquisition of resistance to sorafenib. The study also showed that double blockade of RAF and p38α could be a viable means of overcoming sorafenib resistance [24].

Aberrant Activation of HGF/c-Met Signaling Pathway

Alteration of hepatocyte growth factor (HGF) and its receptor (HGFR; c-met) are implicated in many cancer types, and also associated with poor prognosis and aggressive tumor behavior such as rapid tumor growth, increased angiogenesis and metastasis. HGF/c-met signaling activates MAPK as well as the Akt cascades, which increase cancer cell proliferation and have anti-apoptotic effects on cancer cells, respectively [25]. Previously, a trend toward enhanced survival benefit from sorafenib was reported in patients with low HGF [26]. It is also suggested that c-met copy number may affect the efficiency of sorafenib, at least in vitro [27]. On the other hand, urokinase-type plasminogen activator (uPA) promotes tissue repair through the activation of HGF [28]. Overexpression of uPA and c-met are negative prognostic factors of HCC [29–31]. Induction of miR-193a downregulates uPA, which results in the inhibition of proliferation and induction of apoptosis under conditions of treatment with sorafenib [27]. Similarly, regulators of c-met such as miR-181-5p could reduce invasion of HCC, although the role of miR-181-5p in the effects of sorafenib remains to be clarified [32].

Cellular Response Induced by Hypoxia

It is well known that angiogenesis, which is induced by hypoxia of the tumor tissues, is a primary target of sorafenib. Therefore, angiogenesis and the hypoxia-related cellular response could be promising biomarkers of the antitumor effects of this drug. Several studies have analyzed the association of serum markers related to angiogenesis, such as cytokines and growth factors, with response to sorafenib in HCC. For example, pretreatment level of angiopoietin-2 was correlated with poor response to sorafenib [33]. The alteration of hypoxia-related markers during treatment could be an additional potential marker. Serum levels of des-γ-carboxyprothrombin and lactate dehydrogenase are known to be a surrogate marker of tissue hypoxia and neo-angiogenesis, both of which are associated with the response to sorafenib treatment [34, 35]. Similarly, a decrease of vascular endothelial growth factor was reportedly associated with the longer survival of patients who received sorafenib therapy [36]. On the other hand, a recent report suggests that hypoxia induced by sorafenib increases the stromal-derived factor 1 α (SDF-1α), which activates hepatic satellite cells by binding to C-X-C receptor type 4 (CXCR4) [37]. Blockade of CXCR4 inhibits the tumor fibrosis as well as HCC growth in combination with sorafenib, suggesting that induction of SDF-1α may be involved in the chemoresistance to this drug [37]. It is also reported that galectin-1 is upregulated in the HCC cell line with acquired resistance to sorafenib, and knock down of galectin-1 restores sensitivity [38]. The galectin-1 is under the regulation of Akt/mammalian target of rapamycin/hypoxia-inducible factor-1 pathway; reportedly, it suppresses T cell-mediated cytotoxic immune responses and promotes tumor angiogenesis [39], and is a possible biomarker for predicting response to sorafenib treatment.

Table 1. Previous studies that show potential markers associated with chemoresistance to sorafenib

Potential marker	Description	Materials	References
TGF-β-related			
CD44	HCC cell lines with high expression of CD44 and TGF-β-induced mesenchymal-like phenotype are refractory to sorafenib-induced cell death	Cell lines and xenograft mice model	Fernando et al., 2015
Stress-responsible lncRNA	Stress-responsible lncRNA expression, which is induced by sorafenib, impairs chemotherapy-induced apoptosis	Cell lines	Takahashi et al., 2014
PI3K/Akt-related			
miR-216a/217	miR-216a/217 target PTEN and SMAD7, induce EMT, stem-like properties and acquisition of sorafenib resistance	HCC tissue and cell lines	Xia et al., 2013
RAF/MEK/ERK-related			
miR-122	Survival of miR-122-expressing HCC cells is reduced upon treatment with sorafenib through downregulation of IGF1R	HCC tissue and xenograft mice model	Bai et al., 2009
EGFR and HER-3	In cells with acquired resistance to sorafenib, aberrant activation of EGFR/HER-3 is observed	Xenograft model of mice	Blivet-Van Eggelpoël et al., 2012
JNK and CD133	JNK activation and CD133 expression inversely correlated with the response to sorafenib	HCC tissue	Hagiwara et al., 2012
pERK and Mcl-1	Expressions of pERK and Mcl-1 in HCC before treatment with sorafenib are associated with reduced overall survival	Human HCC tissues	Personeni et al., 2013
FGF-CCND1	HCCs with amplification of FGF-CCND1 locus, including FGF3 and FGF4, showed hypersensitivity to sorafenib	HCC tissue	Arao et al., 2013
NORE1A	NORE1A is identified as a Ras effector and capable of sensitizing cancer cells to sorafenib-induced apoptosis	Cell lines and HCC tissues	Liu et al., 2014
Mapk14 (p38α)	Elevated Mapk14-Atf2 signaling predicts poor response to sorafenib therapy	HCC tissue and xenograft model of mice	Rudalska et al., 2014
miR-224	High miR-224 expression is associated with downregulation of PDGFR and increased survival in HCC patients treated with sorafenib	Serum of HCC patients	Gyöngyösi et al., 2014
HGF-related			
miR-193a	miR-193a is a negative regulator of uPA that promotes the tissue repair through activation of HGF, and a combined treatment with miR-193a and sorafenib inhibit proliferation of HCC cell lines	Cell lines	Salvi et al., 2013
miR-181a-5p	c-Met is a functional target of miR-181a-5p and loss of miR-181a-5p leads to the c-met mediated oncogenic signaling in hepatocarcinogenesis	Cell lines	Korhan et al., 2014
Hypoxia/VEGF-related			
Angiopoietin-2	Serum level of cytokines related to angiogenesis is correlated with poor effects of sorafenib	Serum of HCC patients	Miyahara et al., 2011
DCP	Increase of serum DCP, a surrogate marker of tissue hypoxia, is a predictive marker of tumor response to sorafenib	Serum of HCC patients	Ueshima et al., 2011
LDH	A pre-treatment LDH value, an indirect marker of tumor hypoxia and neo-angiogenesis, is associated with survival of the patients treated with sorafenib	Serum of HCC patients	Faloppi et al., 2014

Table 1. (continued)

Potential marker	Description	Materials	References
VEGF	Decrease of VEGF during treatment is associated with a longer survival of the patients who received sorafenib therapy	Serum of HCC patients	Tsuchiya et al., 2014
SDF-1α/CXCR4	Sorafenib increases SDF-1α expression, and promotes HSC differentiation through SDF-1α/CXCR4 that may be involved in the chemoresistance to sorafenib	Cell lines and mice model	Chen et al., 2014
Galectin-1	The expression of galectin-1 is induced by HIF-1; it suppresses T cell-mediated cytotoxic immune responses and promotes tumor angiogenesis. The overexpression of galectin-1 could be a biomarker of sorafenib resistance	Cell lines	Yeh et al., 2015
Bcl-2 family-related			
Let-7	Let-7c that targets Bcl-xL is downregulated in HCC; expression of let-7c enhances apoptosis of HCC cells treated with sorafenib	HCC tissues and cell lines	Shimizu et al., 2010
Mcl-1	Increased expression of Bcl-2 family protein, Mcl-1, in pretreatment HCC tissues predicts reduced survival of HCC patients treated with sorafenib	HCC tissues	Personeni et al., 2013
miR-34a	miR-34a targets Bcl-2 and potentiates sorafenib-induced apoptosis	Cell lines	Yang et al., 2014
Cancer immunity-related			
NK cell function	Sorafenib inhibits cytotoxicity of NK cells in response to tumor target	Cell lines and mice model	Zhang et al., 2013
miR-1274a	Sorafenib induces miR-1274a through inhibiting ADAM9 and MICA shuddering, which enhances antitumor immunity	Cell lines	Zhou et al., 2011
Teff and Treg	Low dose-sorafenib, but not pharmacologic dose, selectively increases Teff activation while blocking Treg function and enhances antitumor immunity	T cells from HCC patients	Cabrera et al., 2013
Hedgehog signaling and stem cell marker			
Hh signaling	HCC cell lines showing enhanced Hh signaling activity are more resistant to sorafenib	Cell lines	Chen et al., 2011
KRT19	KRT19 knockdown results in decreased resistance to sorafenib	Cell line study	Wilson et al., 2013
EpCAM	EpCAM-enriched cell lines were more resistant to sorafenib	Cell line study	Wilson et al., 2013
Wnt pathway-related			
CTNNB1	Sorafenib attenuates expression of liver-related Wnt-targets, which is accompanied by increased survival of treated mice	HCC tissue and xenograft mice model	Lachenmayer et al., 2012
Genomic instability			
GADD45 β	GADD45 β induction contributes to sorafenib-induced apoptosis in HCC cells	Cell lines	Ou et al., 2010
MCM7	MCM7 expression is correlated with shorter survival after resection and sorafenib inhibited the expression of MCM7	HCC tissue and cell lines	Zhou et al., 2012
Sirtuin 1	Overexpression of Sirtuin 1 promotes tumorigenesis and resistance to sorafenib	HCC tissue and cell lines	Chen et al., 2012

Table 1. (continued)

Potential marker	Description	Materials	References
Tumor suppressive miRs			
miR-425-3p	Higher levels of miR-425-3p are associated with longer survival in HCC patients treated with sorafenib	HCC tissues	Vaira et al., 2015
miR-486	miR-193a inhibits EMT and enhances chemosensitivity of HCC cells to sorafenib through targeting CLDN10 and CITRON	Cell lines	Sun et al., 2015

IGF1R = Insulin-like growth factor type 1 receptor; Mcl-1 = myeloid cell leukemia 1; PDGFR = platelet-derived growth factor receptor; DCP = des-γ-carboxyprothrombin; LDH = lactate dehydrogenase; VEGF = vascular endothelial growth factor; HIF-1 = hypoxia-inducible factor-1; ADAM9 = a disintegrin and metalloproteinase 9; MICA = major histocompatibility complex class-I chain-related protein A; Teff = effector T cell; Treg = regulatory T cell; Hh = Hedgehog; EpCAM = epithelial cell adhesion molecule; CTNNB1 = β-catenin gene; GADD45β = DNA damage-inducible gene 45β; MCM7 = minichromosome maintenance protein 7; CLDN10 = claudin-10; CITRON = rho-interacting, serine/threonine kinase 21 gene.

Activation of Anti-Apoptotic Proteins

The Bcl-2 family consists of pro-apoptotic and anti-apoptotic proteins and is known as a gatekeeper for the apoptotic response. Many kinds of cancer cells show overexpression of anti-apoptotic proteins and downregulation of pro-apoptotic proteins. In HCCs, several reports suggest the role of Bcl-2 family proteins on the acquisition of resistance to sorafenib. MiRs that regulate the expression of the Bcl-2 family may therefore affect the response of HCC to sorafenib. For example, let-7 is downregulated in HCC cell lines, and the putative target of let-7 is Bcl-xL, a known anti-apoptotic protein. In addition, expression of let-7 enhances apoptosis of hepatoma cells upon exposure to sorafenib [40]. Similarly, increased expression of another anti-apoptotic Bcl-2 family protein, myeloid cell leukemia 1, in the pretreatment HCC tissues also predicts reduced overall survival of HCC patients treated with sorafenib [41]. HCC tissues also show reduced expression of miR-34a, which could bind to the 3′-untranslated region of Bcl-2 mRNA and repress its translation. Restoration of miR-34a thus inhibits Bcl-2 expression and potentiates sorafenib-induced apoptosis [42].

Disturbance of Immune Response

As sorafenib is a multi-kinase inhibitor, it may also affect the function of immune cells involved in tumor immunity, which may be associated with treatment response to this drug. The results of a study using a mice model indicate that sorafenib reduces the number of natural killer cells and inhibits the reactivity of natural killer cells through downregulation of its stimulatory receptor [43]. Another report suggested that sorafenib treatment leads to a decrease in effector T cell activation through inhibition of CD25 expression; however, low dose sorafenib restores effector T cell responses by eliminating regulatory T cell suppression [44]. Moreover, sorafenib could induce antitumor immunity by inducing miR-1274a, which regulates a disintegrin and metalloproteinase 9, and by subsequent inhibition of the shedding of major histocompatibility complex class-I [45]. Therefore, immunomodulation induced by sorafenib may be related to drug sensitivity and a combination of immunotherapy with sorafenib could be a promising approach to overcome chemoresistance.

Stem Cell Markers and Hedgehog Signaling Pathway

The expression profiles of stem cell markers, such as epithelial cell adhesion molecule, are reportedly associated with resistance to sorafenib in HCC [46, 47]. Govaere et al. [48] showed that keratin 19 (KRT19)-positive HCC cells also express markers associated with invasion/metastasis as well as hepatic progenitor cell makers, and knockdown of KRT19 results in a decrease of sorafenib resistance in HCC cell lines [48]. It is possible that alterations to cellular signaling induce a proliferative, metastatic and less differentiated expression profile including that of stem cell markers in sorafenib-resistant HCC cells [47]. Chen et al. [49] reported that hedgehog activity was higher in a subset of HCC cell lines with EMT phenotype that were reportedly more resistant to sorafenib.

Others

A recent report showed that activation of the Wnt pathway can be divided into 2 types according to the profile of dysregulated Wnt target molecules. A subset of

HCCs characterized by the upregulation of liver-specific Wnt targets, nuclear staining of TGF-β, expression of glutamine synthetase and enrichment of CTNNB1 mutation were sensitive to sorafenib [50]. Similarly, DNA damage-inducible gene *45β* is more predominantly expressed in HCC cells that are sensitive to sorafenib treatment [51]. Dysregulation of minichromosome maintenance protein 7 is a predictor of the prognosis of HCC patients, and sorafenib inhibits its expression [52]. Overexpression of the NAD+-dependent histone deacetylases, Sirtuin 1, is detected in HCCs with a higher tumor grade and is associated with poor survival as well as resistance to sorafenib [53]. Finally, expression of miRs that are considered to have tumor suppressor functions, such as miR-425-3p and miR-486, may also predict the effect of sorafenib [54, 55]. Given the fact that a single miR targets multiple kinds of mRNA, constitutive activation of multiple molecules may act in concert to restore the sensitivity of HCC to sorafenib [56]. Studies on molecular biology and signal transduction are a key issue to understanding the efficacy of systemic therapy to HCC [57–60].

Conclusion

In this review, we focused on the molecular mechanism of chemoresistance to sorafenib in HCC and summarized the recent reports, which was listed in table 1. So far, sorafenib is the only drug that improves survival in advanced HCC [61, 62]. Therefore, understanding and overcoming chemoresistance to this drug is critical for the improvement of survival in patients with advanced HCC. It is possible that multiple signaling pathways are involved in the acquisition of resistance [57–60]. Recent intensive studies will provide critical information regarding combination therapy with sorafenib that could form the basis of personalized medicine for this refractory cancer.

Acknowledgments

This work was supported in part by Grant-in-Aid for Scientific Research (KAKENHI: 24590997) from the Japanese Society for the Promotion of Science (N.N.), a grant from the Smoking Research Foundation (N.N.) and a grand from the Japan Health Foundation (N.N.).

Author Contributions

N.N. drafted the manuscript and wrote the final version. M.K., T.S. and M.K. approved the final version of the manuscript.

Disclosure Statement

The authors have no conflicts of interest to disclose.

References

1 Torre LA, Bray F, Siegel RL, Ferlay J, Lortet-Tieulent J, Jemal A: Global cancer statistics, 2012. CA Cancer J Clin 2015;65:87–108.

2 Kudo M: Treatment of advanced hepatocellular carcinoma with emphasis on hepatic arterial infusion chemotherapy and molecular targeted therapy. Liver Cancer 2012;1:62–70.

3 Llovet JM, Ricci S, Mazzaferro V, Hilgard P, Gane E, Blanc JF, de Oliveira AC, Santoro A, Raoul JL, Forner A, Schwartz M, Porta C, Zeuzem S, Bolondi L, Greten TF, Galle PR, Seitz JF, Borbath I, Häussinger D, Giannaris T, Shan M, Moscovici M, Voliotis D, Bruix J; SHARP Investigators Study Group: Sorafenib in advanced hepatocellular carcinoma. N Engl J Med 2008;359:378–390.

4 Kudo M: Biomarkers and personalized sorafenib therapy. Liver Cancer 2014;3:399–404.

5 Shao YY, Hsu CH, Cheng AL: Predictive biomarkers of antiangiogenic therapy for advanced hepatocellular carcinoma: where are we? Liver Cancer 2013;2:93–107.

6 Fernando J, Malfettone A, Cepeda EB, Vilarrasa-Blasi R, Bertran E, Raimondi G, Fabra À, Alvarez-Barrientos A, Fernández-Salguero P, Fernández-Rodríguez CM, Giannelli G, Sancho P, Fabregat I: A mesenchymal-like phenotype and expression of CD44 predict lack of apoptotic response to sorafenib in liver tumor cells. Int J Cancer 2015;136:E161–E172.

7 Takahashi K, Yan IK, Kogure T, Haga H, Patel T: Extracellular vesicle-mediated transfer of long non-coding RNA ROR modulates chemosensitivity in human hepatocellular cancer. FEBS Open Bio 2014;4:458–467.

8 Xia H, Ooi LL, Hui KM: MicroRNA-216a/217-induced epithelial-mesenchymal transition targets PTEN and SMAD7 to promote drug resistance and recurrence of liver cancer. Hepatology 2013;58:629–641.

9 Liu L, Cao Y, Chen C, Zhang X, McNabola A, Wilkie D, Wilhelm S, Lynch M, Carter C: Sorafenib blocks the RAF/MEK/ERK pathway, inhibits tumor angiogenesis, and induces tumor cell apoptosis in hepatocellular carcinoma model PLC/PRF/5. Cancer Res 2006;66:11851–11858.

10 Nishida N, Kudo M: Recent advancements in comprehensive genetic analyses for human hepatocellular carcinoma. Oncology 2013;84(suppl 1):93–97.

11 Nishida N, Fukuda Y, Komeda T, Kita R, Sando T, Furukawa M, Amenomori M, Shibagaki I, Nakao K, Ikenaga M, et al: Amplification and overexpression of the cyclin D1 gene in aggressive human hepatocellular carcinoma. Cancer Res 1994;54:3107–3110.

12 Arao T, Ueshima K, Matsumoto K, Nagai T, Kimura H, Hagiwara S, Sakurai T, Haji S, Kanazawa A, Hidaka H, Iso Y, Kubota K, Shimada M, Utsunomiya T, Hirooka M, Hiasa Y, Toyoki Y, Hakamada K, Yasui K, Kumada T, Toyoda H, Sato S, Hisai H, Kuzuya T, Tsuchiya K, Izumi N, Arii S, Nishio K, Kudo M: FGF3/FGF4 amplification and multiple lung metastases in responders to sorafenib in hepatocellular carcinoma. Hepatology 2013;57:1407–1415.

13 Schulze K, Imbeaud S, Letouze E, Alexandrov LB, Calderaro J, Rebouissou S, Couchy G, Meiller C, Shinde J, Soysouvanh F, Calatayud AL, Pinyol R, Pelletier L, Balabaud C, Laurent A, Blanc JF, Mazzaferro V, Calvo F, Villanueva A, Nault JC, Bioulac-Sage P, Stratton MR, Llovet JM, Zucman-Rossi J: Exome sequencing of hepatocellular carcinomas identifies new mutational signatures and potential therapeutic targets. Nat Genet 2015;47:505–511.
14 Nishida N, Nishimura T, Nagasaka T, Ikai I, Goel A, Boland CR: Extensive methylation is associated with beta-catenin mutations in hepatocellular carcinoma: evidence for two distinct pathways of human hepatocarcinogenesis. Cancer Res 2007;67:4586–4594.
15 Nishida N, Nagasaka T, Nishimura T, Ikai I, Boland CR, Goel A: Aberrant methylation of multiple tumor suppressor genes in aging liver, chronic hepatitis, and hepatocellular carcinoma. Hepatology 2008;47:908–918.
16 Nishida N, Kudo M, Nagasaka T, Ikai I, Goel A: Characteristic patterns of altered DNA methylation predict emergence of human hepatocellular carcinoma. Hepatology 2012;56: 994–1003.
17 Nishida N, Kudo M: Oxidative stress and epigenetic instability in human hepatocarcinogenesis. Dig Dis 2013;31:447–453.
18 Liu LL, Zhang MF, Pan YH, Yun JP, Zhang CZ: NORE1A sensitises cancer cells to sorafenib-induced apoptosis and indicates hepatocellular carcinoma prognosis. Tumour Biol 2014;35:1763–1774.
19 Nishida N, Nishimura T, Nakai T, Chishina H, Arizumi T, Takita M, Kitai S, Yada N, Hagiwara S, Inoue T, Minami Y, Ueshima K, Sakurai T, Kudo M: Genome-wide profiling of DNA methylation and tumor progression in human hepatocellular carcinoma. Dig Dis 2014;32:658–663.
20 Bai S, Nasser MW, Wang B, Hsu SH, Datta J, Kutay H, Yadav A, Nuovo G, Kumar P, Ghoshal K: MicroRNA-122 inhibits tumorigenic properties of hepatocellular carcinoma cells and sensitizes these cells to sorafenib. J Biol Chem 2009;284:32015–32027.
21 Gyöngyösi B, Végh E, Járay B, Székely E, Fassan M, Bodoky G, Schaff Z, Kiss A: Pretreatment microRNA level and outcome in sorafenib-treated hepatocellular carcinoma. J Histochem Cytochem 2014;62:547–555.
22 Blivet-Van Eggelpoël MJ, Chettouh H, Fartoux L, Aoudjehane L, Barbu V, Rey C, Priam S, Housset C, Rosmorduc O, Desbois-Mouthon C: Epidermal growth factor receptor and HER-3 restrict cell response to sorafenib in hepatocellular carcinoma cells. J Hepatol 2012;57:108–115.
23 Hagiwara S, Kudo M, Nagai T, Inoue T, Ueshima K, Nishida N, Watanabe T, Sakurai T: Activation of JNK and high expression level of CD133 predict a poor response to sorafenib in hepatocellular carcinoma. Br J Cancer 2012;106:1997–2003.
24 Rudalska R, Dauch D, Longerich T, McJunkin K, Wuestefeld T, Kang TW, Hohmeyer A, Pesic M, Leibold J, von Thun A, Schirmacher P, Zuber J, Weiss KH, Powers S, Malek NP, Eilers M, Sipos B, Lowe SW, Geffers R, Laufer S, Zender L: In vivo RNAi screening identifies a mechanism of sorafenib resistance in liver cancer. Nat Med 2014;20:1138–1146.
25 Xiao GH, Jeffers M, Bellacosa A, Mitsuuchi Y, Vande Woude GF, Testa JR: Anti-apoptotic signaling by hepatocyte growth factor/Met via the phosphatidylinositol 3-kinase/Akt and mitogen-activated protein kinase pathways. Proc Natl Acad Sci U S A 2001;98:247–252.
26 Llovet JM, Peña CE, Lathia CD, Shan M, Meinhardt G, Bruix J; SHARP Investigators Study Group: Plasma biomarkers as predictors of outcome in patients with advanced hepatocellular carcinoma. Clin Cancer Res 2012;18:2290–2300.
27 Salvi A, Conde I, Abeni E, Arici B, Grossi I, Specchia C, Portolani N, Barlati S, De Petro G: Effects of miR-193a and sorafenib on hepatocellular carcinoma cells. Mol Cancer 2013;12: 162.
28 Sisson TH, Nguyen MH, Yu B, Novak ML, Simon RH, Koh TJ: Urokinase-type plasminogen activator increases hepatocyte growth factor activity required for skeletal muscle regeneration. Blood 2009;114:5052–5061.
29 Tavian D, De Petro G, Benetti A, Portolani N, Giulini SM, Barlati S: u-PA and c-MET mRNA expression is co-ordinately enhanced while hepatocyte growth factor mRNA is down-regulated in human hepatocellular carcinoma. Int J Cancer 2000;87:644–649.
30 Salvi A, Arici B, De Petro G, Barlati S: Small interfering RNA urokinase silencing inhibits invasion and migration of human hepatocellular carcinoma cells. Mol Cancer Ther 2004; 3:671–678.
31 Salvi A, Arici B, Portolani N, Giulini SM, De Petro G, Barlati S: In vitro c-met inhibition by antisense RNA and plasmid-based RNAi down-modulates migration and invasion of hepatocellular carcinoma cells. Int J Oncol 2007;31:451–460.
32 Korhan P, Erdal E, Atabey N: MiR-181a-5p is downregulated in hepatocellular carcinoma and suppresses motility, invasion and branching-morphogenesis by directly targeting c-Met. Biochem Biophys Res Commun 2014;450:1304–1312.
33 Miyahara K, Nouso K, Tomoda T, Kobayashi S, Hagihara H, Kuwaki K, Toshimori J, Onishi H, Ikeda F, Miyake Y, Nakamura S, Shiraha H, Takaki A, Yamamoto K: Predicting the treatment effect of sorafenib using serum angiogenesis markers in patients with hepatocellular carcinoma. J Gastroenterol Hepatol 2011;26:1604–1611.
34 Ueshima K, Kudo M, Takita M, Nagai T, Tatsumi C, Ueda T, Kitai S, Ishikawa E, Yada N, Inoue T, Hagiwara S, Minami Y, Chung H, Sakurai T: Des-γ-carboxyprothrombin may be a promising biomarker to determine the therapeutic efficacy of sorafenib for hepatocellular carcinoma. Dig Dis 2011;29:321–325.
35 Faloppi L, Scartozzi M, Bianconi M, Svegliati Baroni G, Toniutto P, Giampieri R, Del Prete M, De Minicis S, Bitetto D, Loretelli C, D'Anzeo M, Benedetti A, Cascinu S: The role of LDH serum levels in predicting global outcome in HCC patients treated with sorafenib: implications for clinical management. BMC Cancer 2014;14:110.
36 Tsuchiya K, Asahina Y, Matsuda S, Muraoka M, Nakata T, Suzuki Y, Tamaki N, Yasui Y, Suzuki S, Hosokawa T, Nishimura T, Ueda K, Kuzuya T, Nakanishi H, Itakura J, Takahashi Y, Kurosaki M, Enomoto N, Izumi N: Changes in plasma vascular endothelial growth factor at 8 weeks after sorafenib administration as predictors of survival for advanced hepatocellular carcinoma. Cancer 2014;120:229–237.
37 Chen Y, Huang Y, Reiberger T, Duyverman AM, Huang P, Samuel R, Hiddingh L, Roberge S, Koppel C, Lauwers GY, Zhu AX, Jain RK, Duda DG: Differential effects of sorafenib on liver versus tumor fibrosis mediated by stromal-derived factor 1 alpha/C-X-C receptor type 4 axis and myeloid differentiation antigen-positive myeloid cell infiltration in mice. Hepatology 2014;59:1435–1447.
38 Yeh CC, Hsu CH, Shao YY, Ho WC, Tsai MH, Feng WC, Chow LP: Integrated stable isotope labeling by amino acids in cell culture (SILAC) and isobaric tags for relative and absolute quantitation (iTRAQ) quantitative proteomic analysis identifies galectin-1 as a potential biomarker for predicting sorafenib resistance in liver cancer. Mol Cell Proteomics 2015;14:1527–1545.
39 Ito K, Stannard K, Gabutero E, Clark AM, Neo SY, Onturk S, Blanchard H, Ralph SJ: Galectin-1 as a potent target for cancer therapy: role in the tumor microenvironment. Cancer Metastasis Rev 2012;31:763–778.
40 Shimizu S, Takehara T, Hikita H, Kodama T, Miyagi T, Hosui A, Tatsumi T, Ishida H, Noda T, Nagano H, Doki Y, Mori M, Hayashi N: The let-7 family of microRNAs inhibits Bcl-xL expression and potentiates sorafenib-induced apoptosis in human hepatocellular carcinoma. J Hepatol 2010;52:698–704.
41 Personeni N, Rimassa L, Pressiani T, Destro A, Ligorio C, Tronconi MC, Bozzarelli S, Carnaghi C, Di Tommaso L, Giordano L, Roncalli M, Santoro A: Molecular determinants of outcome in sorafenib-treated patients with hepatocellular carcinoma. J Cancer Res Clin Oncol 2013;139:1179–1187.
42 Yang F, Li QJ, Gong ZB, Zhou L, You N, Wang S, Li XL, Li JJ, An JZ, Wang DS, He Y, Dou KF: MicroRNA-34a targets Bcl-2 and sensitizes human hepatocellular carcinoma cells to sorafenib treatment. Technol Cancer Res Treat 2014;13:77–86.
43 Zhang QB, Sun HC, Zhang KZ, Jia QA, Bu Y, Wang M, Chai ZT, Zhang QB, Wang WQ, Kong LQ, Zhu XD, Lu L, Wu WZ, Wang L, Tang ZY: Suppression of natural killer cells by sorafenib contributes to prometastatic effects in hepatocellular carcinoma. PLoS One 2013; 8:e55945.

44 Cabrera R, Ararat M, Xu Y, Brusko T, Wasserfall C, Atkinson MA, Chang LJ, Liu C, Nelson DR: Immune modulation of effector CD4+ and regulatory T cell function by sorafenib in patients with hepatocellular carcinoma. Cancer Immunol Immunother 2013; 62:737–746.

45 Zhou C, Liu J, Li Y, Liu L, Zhang X, Ma CY, Hua SC, Yang M, Yuan Q: microRNA-1274a, a modulator of sorafenib induced a disintegrin and metalloproteinase 9 (ADAM9) downregulation in hepatocellular carcinoma. FEBS Lett 2011;585:1828–1834.

46 Wilson GS, Hu Z, Duan W, Tian A, Wang XM, McLeod D, Lam V, George J, Qiao L: Efficacy of using cancer stem cell markers in isolating and characterizing liver cancer stem cells. Stem Cells Dev 2013;22:2655–2664.

47 Xin HW, Ambe CM, Hari DM, Wiegand GW, Miller TC, Chen JQ, Anderson AJ, Ray S, Mullinax JE, Koizumi T, Langan RC, Burka D, Herrmann MA, Goldsmith PK, Stojadinovic A, Rudloff U, Thorgeirsson SS, Avital I: Label-retaining liver cancer cells are relatively resistant to sorafenib. Gut 2013;62:1777–1786.

48 Govaere O, Komuta M, Berkers J, Spee B, Janssen C, de Luca F, Katoonizadeh A, Wouters J, van Kempen LC, Durnez A, Verslype C, De Kock J, Rogiers V, van Grunsven LA, Topal B, Pirenne J, Vankelecom H, Nevens F, van den Oord J, Pinzani M, Roskams T: Keratin 19: a key role player in the invasion of human hepatocellular carcinomas. Gut 2014;63:674–685.

49 Chen X, Lingala S, Khoobyari S, Nolta J, Zern MA, Wu J: Epithelial mesenchymal transition and hedgehog signaling activation are associated with chemoresistance and invasion of hepatoma subpopulations. J Hepatol 2011;55: 838–845.

50 Lachenmayer A, Alsinet C, Savic R, Cabellos L, Toffanin S, Hoshida Y, Villanueva A, Minguez B, Newell P, Tsai HW, Barretina J, Thung S, Ward SC, Bruix J, Mazzaferro V, Schwartz M, Friedman SL, Llovet JM: Wnt-pathway activation in two molecular classes of hepatocellular carcinoma and experimental modulation by sorafenib. Clin Cancer Res 2012;18:4997–5007.

51 Ou DL, Shen YC, Yu SL, Chen KF, Yeh PY, Fan HH, Feng WC, Wang CT, Lin LI, Hsu C, Cheng AL: Induction of DNA damage-inducible gene GADD45beta contributes to sorafenib-induced apoptosis in hepatocellular carcinoma cells. Cancer Res 2010;70: 9309–9318.

52 Zhou YM, Zhang XF, Cao L, Li B, Sui CJ, Li YM, Yin ZF: MCM7 expression predicts post-operative prognosis for hepatocellular carcinoma. Liver Int 2012;32:1505–1509.

53 Chen HC, Jeng YM, Yuan RH, Hsu HC, Chen YL: SIRT1 promotes tumorigenesis and resistance to chemotherapy in hepatocellular carcinoma and its expression predicts poor prognosis. Ann Surg Oncol 2012;19:2011–2019.

54 Vaira V, Roncalli M, Carnaghi C, Faversani A, Maggioni M, Augello C, Rimassa L, Pressiani T, Spagnuolo G, Di Tommaso L, Fagiuoli S, Rota Caremoli E, Barberis M, Labianca R, Santoro A, Bosari S: MicroRNA-425-3p predicts response to sorafenib therapy in patients with hepatocellular carcinoma. Liver Int 2015;35:1077–1086.

55 Sun H, Cui C, Xiao F, Wang H, Xu J, Shi X, Yang Y, Zhang Q, Zheng X, Yang X, Wu C, Wang L: miR-486 regulates metastasis and chemosensitivity in hepatocellular carcinoma by targeting CLDN10 and CITRON. Hepatol Res 2015, Epub ahead of print.

56 Peveling-Oberhag J, Döring C, Hartmann S, Filmann N, Mertens A, Piiper A, Herrmann E, Hansmann ML, Zeuzem S, Trojan J, Welker MW: Feasibility of global miRNA analysis from fine-needle biopsy FFPE material in patients with hepatocellular carcinoma treated with sorafenib. Clin Sci(Lond) 2015;128:29–37.

57 Sakurai T, Kudo M: Molecular link between liver fibrosis and hepatocellular carcinoma. Liver Cancer 2013;2:365–366.

58 Ramakrishna G, Rastogi A, Trehanpati N, Sen B, Khosla R, Sarin SK: From cirrhosis to hepatocellular carcinoma: new molecular insights on inflammation and cellular senescence. Liver Cancer 2013;2:367–383.

59 Nishida N, Kudo M: Alteration of epigenetic profile in human hepatocellular carcinoma and its clinical implications. Liver Cancer 2014;3:417–427.

60 Effendi K, Yamazaki K, Fukuma M, Sakamoto M: Overexpression of leucine-rich repeat-containing G protein-coupled receptor 5 (LGR5) represents a typical Wnt/β-catenin pathway-activated hepatocellular carcinoma. Liver Cancer 2014;3:451–457.

61 Lachenmayer A, Alsinet C, Chang CY, Llovet JM: Molecular approaches to treatment of hepatocellular carcinoma. Dig Liver Dis 2010; 42(suppl 3):S264–S272.

62 Kudo M: Why does every hepatocellular carcinoma clinical trial using molecular targeted agents fail? Liver Cancer 2012;1:59–60.

Review Article

Digestive Diseases

Dig Dis 2015;33:780–790
DOI: 10.1159/000439103

Challenges of Clinical Research on Hepatocellular Carcinoma

Masatoshi Kudo Masayuki Kitano Toshiharu Sakurai Naoshi Nishida

Department of Gastroenterology and Hepatology, Kinki University School of Medicine, Osaka-Sayama, Osaka, Japan

Key Words
Hepatocellular carcinoma · Clinical research · Prospective randomized clinical trial · Diagnosis · Treatment

Abstract
Challenges of clinical practice and research on hepatocellular carcinoma (HCC) were reviewed. There are several differences in clinical practice between Japan and the Western countries such as tumor markers, understanding of pathological early HCC, imaging diagnosis, treatment strategy, staging system and subclassification of HCC. Further studies are warranted for the clinical practices of Japan to be adopted in the rest of the world.

Introduction

Many diagnostic and treatment techniques for hepatocellular carcinoma (HCC) that are at the global forefront have been developed in Japan. In particular, progress in clinical research on HCC made by Japanese researchers has been introduced to the world via peer-reviewed medical and science journals. Yet, many issues remain to be addressed. This article discusses the current situation, recent progress [1], remaining challenges and future prospects of clinical investigations on HCC.

Tumor Markers

Tumor markers are routinely used in screening, diagnosis, treatment response evaluation, assessment of tumor malignancy and diagnosis of tumor recurrence, and among them, alpha-fetoprotein (AFP) has long been appreciated as a tumor marker for HCC. In Japan, prothrombin induced by vitamin K absence-II (PIVKA-II), and the L3 fraction of AFP (AFP-L3) [2–4] are routinely used alongside AFP to screen for HCC. However, in other countries, the clinical guidelines for HCC, such as those issued by the American Association for the Study of Liver Diseases (AASLD) [5] and the European Association for the Study of the Liver (EASL) [6], do not recommend the use of PIVKA-II or AFP-L3 in daily clinical practice. Even AFP is not recommended for the surveillance of liver cancer because of its low sensitivity and specificity, that is, due to its poor cost effectiveness, leaving ultrasound (US) as the only screening method recommended per the Western guidelines [7]. This signifies a huge difference in the way of thinking between researchers in Japan and those in Western countries. In Japan, all of these 3 tumor markers are fully covered by the National Health Insurance System, and an increase in any of them when used in combination can lead to the detection and diagnosis of small HCC. From this perspective, it is important to perform prospective clinical trials to demonstrate that the regular use of tumor markers, including AFP, is an essential part of liver

Masatoshi Kudo, MD, PhD
Department of Gastroenterology and Hepatology
Kinki University School of Medicine, 377-2 Ohno-Higashi
Osaka-Sayama, Osaka 589-8511 (Japan)
E-Mail m-kudo@med.kindai.ac.jp

cancer screening. For this purpose, a clinical trial headed by the University of Tokyo for HCC, the ALDUS Study, is currently ongoing and its results are eagerly awaited.

AFP has numerous future roles. Both AFP levels and HCC incidence decrease markedly when a sustained virologic response (SVR) is achieved by the eradication of hepatitis C virus by interferon (IFN) therapy for chronic hepatitis C. However, it is unclear whether this reduction in AFP reflects improvement of the inflammation or of the background liver tissue that served as the primary origin. According to Asahina et al. [8], the rate of hepatocarcinogenesis is low in SVR patients when AFP level is <6 ng/ml, but is high in patients with AFP ≥6 ng/ml even after they have achieved SVR. It has also been reported that post-SVR carcinogenesis rates vary among hepatitis C patients with AFP levels lesser or higher than 10 ng/ml [9]. On the basis of these reports, AFP is used as a surrogate marker for carcinogenesis in SVR patients after antiviral therapy for hepatitis C. Although IFN-free antiviral therapy with direct acting antivirals (DAAs) is expected to become the mainstream therapy for chronic hepatitis C, it is currently unclear whether the suppression of carcinogenesis is similar between patients who have achieved SVR after taking DAA agents that act directly on the virus and those who achieved SVR after receiving IFN-based therapy, which exerts antitumor and immunostimulatory effects. It becomes clear that an all-oral DAA regimen can decrease AFP levels that serve as an indicator. However, it is not clear whether low-dose long-term IFN therapy can decrease AFP levels in SVR patients with AFP ≥6 ng/ml after DAA therapy. It seems, then, that AFP in both its conventional and newer uses has clear prospects for the future, but certain challenges such as those mentioned above are yet to be addressed.

PIVKA-II, which is an independent marker for HCC and has no correlation with AFP, is also used in screening, treatment response evaluation [10], diagnosis of recurrent HCC and assessment of biological malignancy grade. The association between PIVKA-II level and vascular invasion is of particular interest. According to Koike et al. [11], patients with high PIVKA-II levels have a high incidence of portal invasion. Vascular invasion, however, is suppressed by the administration of vitamin K, which downregulates PIVKA-II. This evidence prompted a large-scale clinical trial to investigate whether Vitamin K suppresses the recurrence of HCC in patients who received curative treatment such as resection [12, 13] or ablation [14, 15]. The study was unsuccessful though, and it completely ruled out the possibility of vitamin K for tertiary prevention after curative treatment of HCC [16]. PIVKA-II levels are also known to increase during treatment more often in patients who respond to sorafenib, a molecular targeted agent, suggesting that PIVKA-II can serve as a surrogate marker for the suppression of angiogenesis or as an indicator of treatment response [17]. This possibility needs to be investigated further in systemic therapy [18, 19].

AFP-L3 does not correlate with AFP or PIVKA-II in patients with HCC [2, 4]. In recent years, the measurement of highly sensitive AFP-L3 has been attracting attention because this innovative method enables AFP-L3 to be measured even when total AFP levels are ≤10 ng/ml. Compared with conventional AFP-L3, highly sensitive AFP-L3 has a high positive rate even in patients with early-stage HCCs (e.g. stages I and II), making the marker useful in the early diagnosis of HCC [20, 21]. The malignancy rate of AFP-L3–positive liver cancer is extremely high, and while the survival of AFP-L3–negative patients who had high AFP-L3 levels before treatment is similar to the survival of patients negative for AFP-L3 throughout treatment, and the survival of patients who maintain high AFP-L3 levels even after treatment is significantly poor [4, 22].

As we gain a more comprehensive understanding of these markers' characteristics, it is likely that AFP, PIVKA-II and AFP-L3 will be increasingly used for prognostic prediction and assessment of the biological malignancy. In addition, we need to report actively on the utility of PIVKA-II and AFP-L3 to the world, especially the United States and Europe where use of these 2 markers is not recommended in their guidelines [7].

Diagnosis

Ultrasonography

Guidelines published all over the world recommend B-mode US as a first-line imaging modality for screening HCC. However, when B-mode US is used to screen patients with cirrhosis, small liver tumors are often overlooked because of coarse liver parenchyma. Although US is the only screening modality recommended in the guidelines issued by the AASLD [5], the EASL [6] and the Asian Pacific Association for the Study of the Liver (APASL) [23], in Japan, both sets of guidelines – the Evidence-based Clinical Practice Guidelines [24] and the Consensus-based Clinical Practice Guidelines [25] – recommend annual or semiannual computed tomography (CT) or magnetic resonance imaging (MRI) for type B or C cirrhotic patients, who have very high risk for liver cancer, due to the inherent limitations of B-mode US.

Dig Dis 2015;33:780–790
DOI: 10.1159/000439103

Sonazoid-enhanced US, which is composed of the vascular phase and Kupffer phase, has recently been used proactively for screening as well as diagnosis of liver cancer [26, 27]. Perfusion defects can be detected easily in the Kupffer phase, which starts 10 min after venous injection. HCC can be accurately diagnosed by performing US after the re-injection of sonazoid [26, 28]. This was verified in a multicenter randomized clinical trial (NCT No. 00822991), and thus, it is highly likely that surveillance using Kupffer phase imaging in Sonazoid-enhanced US will be recommended in future editions of clinical practice guidelines for HCC.

Elastography is also now frequently performed to diagnose fibrosis in patients with diffuse liver disease. Elastography is simply classified by the measurement method used, namely, strain elastography or shear wave elastography (SWE). The representative strain method, real-time elastography (RTE), simplifies the diagnosis of fibrosis with the use of a liver fibrosis index [29]. Representative shear wave methods are FibroScan (transient elastography), virtual touch quantification and SWE, and they determine the stiffness of the liver by generating push pulses in order to measure the propagating shear waves. FibroScan is particularly well known for enabling liver cancer risk to be judged from liver stiffness measurements in patients with type B or C cirrhosis [30–32]. Consequently, FibroScan is a highly useful method for predicting the risk for cancer without an invasive biopsy, but it remains to be confirmed whether shear wave methods and RTE can produce results as good as FibroScan.

CT

Multidetector raw CT is the mainstream CT procedure that is in use today [33]. Further research is needed to reveal the utility of effective hepatic parenchymal blood flow by perfusion CT, as well as liver function assessment by dual energy CT.

MRI

A recent MRI-related topic attracting attention is the approval of gadolinium ethoxybenzyl diethylenetriamine pentaacetic acid-enhanced MRI (EOB-MRI). Early HCCs demonstrating hypovascularity on CT during hepatic arteriography (CTHA) or no decrease in portal flow on CT during arterial portography (CTAP) may be detected as hypointense signals on EOB-MRI [34, 35]. Such hypointense nodules are often diagnosed histopathologically as early HCCs [25, 36, 37]. Although there has been a report of dysplastic nodules occasionally displaying hypointensity even in the hepatocyte phase of EOB-MRI, such results were just based on a comparison with liver biopsy and EOB-MRI findings. In fact, a study that followed the natural course of hypointense hypovascular nodules has revealed that such nodules most likely develop into classical hypervascular HCC [38–56]. On the other hand, some early HCC nodules may not show hypointensity in the hepatocyte phase of EOB-MRI. More follow-up studies are needed to clarify this issue.

Another interesting topic concerning EOB-MRI is the role of transporters in HCC. The transporter that imports EOB into the hepatocytes is an organic anion transporting polypeptide 8 (OATP8 or OATP1B3) [57, 58]. Patients with typical moderately differentiated HCC that displays hyperintensity in the hepatocyte phase of EOB-MRI account for 5–10% of all HCC patients. Furthermore, OATP8-positive liver cancers are reported to be a subtype of HCC and exhibit a benign nature [59, 60]. In studies by Yoneda et al. [61] and Yamashita et al. [62], the expression of β-catenin is significantly upregulated in HCC expressing OATP8, suggesting that OATP8 is induced by Wnt/β-catenin signaling. Yamashita et al. [63] also recently revealed that the expression of OATP8 is inhibited by the transcription factor hepatocyte nuclear factor 4A and that OATP8-positive HCC is a subtype of HCC that expresses a specific group of genes. These findings suggest that EOB-MRI is a molecular imaging modality that acutely reflects the expression of OATP8 and will be useful for the assessment of multistep carcinogenesis in liver cancer [58] and the identification of benign HCC subtypes. Further studies are needed to confirm this proposal.

Angiography

Recent advances in CT, contrast-US and EOB-MRI have meant that angiography is no longer necessary diagnostically as it was in the past. However, CTHA and CTAP still play extremely important roles in the detection of small HCC and in the differentiation from liver shunt. An extremely important angiographic finding is that when patients with hypervascular HCC undergo single-level dynamic CTHA, the contrast agent injected via the hepatic artery stains hypervascular HCC intensely and then drains from the tumor capsule to stain the surrounding liver tissue in a corona-like fashion [64]. Such corona-like staining is also observed in dynamic CT after careful examination, making this dynamic CT finding important for differentiating HCC from other tumors [65]. It is anticipated that CTHA and CTAP will be used more often in treatment to monitor the degree of lipiodol retention during transcatheter arterial chemoembolization (TACE), although this is not absolutely necessary in routine clinical practice. In fact, it should be sufficient in daily clinical practice to perform dynamic CT, Sonazoid-enhanced US and EOB-MRI.

Treatment

Hepatectomy

Hepatectomy is the one of the curative treatment modalities [12]. A recent popular topic related to hepatectomy is the usefulness of intraoperative US [66] and the intravenous administration of oral indocyanine green (ICG) before surgery. ICG accumulation within the HCC tumor helps to localize the liver cancer. This technique, the so-called 'ICG fluorescence imaging', enables the detection of small intrahepatic metastases that are just a few millimeters in size and therefore not detected preoperatively [67]. However, the problem associated with ICG fluorescence imaging is that only tumors near the liver surface are detected because the near-infrared fluorescence of ICG is transmitted just 5–10 mm from the liver surface. Although the exact mechanism of ICG uptake by HCC remains to be elucidated, the accumulation of ICG in HCC, but not in non-cancerous liver tissue, may be not only due to the presence of ICG uptake transporters in HCC but also due to some defect in ICG excretion transporters. The future challenges associated with hepatectomy include how to detect lesions deep inside the liver and how to apply ICG fluorescence imaging in laparoscopic surgery.

Recent technical advances have made laparoscopic hepatectomy an easy and favored technique due to its minimally invasive nature [68, 69]. When performed for small HCCs located in laparoscopically accessible areas, laparoscopic hepatectomy minimizes blood loss, shortens operation time and hospital stay and offers good long-term prognosis comparable with laparotomic hepatectomy. It is, therefore, likely that the use of laparoscopic hepatectomy will become more widespread as a minimally invasive surgical procedure.

Adjuvant therapy after curative resection is also a challenging issue [70]. Another challenging issue in Japan is a transplantation [71–73]. Only living donor liver transplantation is performed in Japan.

Locoregional Therapy

Locoregional therapy has evolved from ethanol injection to microwave ablation and then to radiofrequency ablation (RFA). Today, RFA accounts for approximately 99% of all locoregional therapies that are being undertaken. The latest development in RFA treatments for HCC is the application of Celon electrodes that allows for expansion of the ablation area, owing to the bipolar needle electrodes used. Treatment is possible without touching the tumor because 2 needle punctures are made. Since the bipolar electrodes require no return electrode, they are also associated with low risks of burn and damage to surrounding organs. Clear advantages of using needle electrodes are, therefore, the non-touch ablation of tumor tissue due to the placement of 2 electrodes and also, unlike conventional overlapping ablation, the ability to avoid reduced puncture accuracy because the tumor is punctured with multiple electrodes prior to thermal coagulation. Consequently, this method of locoregional therapy is expected to become popular, although it remains to be seen whether bipolar needle electrodes replace the conventional Cool-tip® needles used.

Other developments in RFA include the application of contrast-enhanced US, fusion imaging using volume data from CT, MRI and US and fusion imaging combined with contrast-enhanced US to treat lesions that are not detectable with B-mode US. Although any of these imaging options can be used to help localize tumors precisely and insert needle electrodes, fusion imaging is particularly useful for the determination of accurate ablative margins [69].

The injection of lipiodol before RFA is extremely useful in confirming the ablative margins. Without lipiodol injection, it is impossible to determine accurate ablative margins by simple comparison of pre- and post-ablation images placed side by side in the display. This is why the pre-treatment injection of lipiodol was mandatory in the past, even though it requires an angiographic procedure before RFA. Today, fusion images before and after RFA can be overlaid using an extracted overlay method [74]. However, the method needs to be improved further because it currently involves cumbersome procedures including using the workstation.

TACE

Recent advances in TACE include the development of microsphere embolic agents. In Japan, conventional TACE (cTACE) [75, 76] is routinely performed to inject a liquid containing an antitumor agent via the hepatic artery, which is followed by embolization with gelatin sponge particles. However, the introduction of microspheres such as DC Beads®, HepaSphere and Embosphere in 2014 has increased the treatment options related to TACE. Therefore, the challenge today is in the selection of different beads for TACE, also known as drug eluting beads TACE (DEB-TACE) and cTACE. Microsphere beads of exactly the same size embolize blood vessels of a certain diameter, and their advantages are their non-absorbent property and excellent biocompatibility, thus rarely causing inflammatory reactions in the body. The microsphere beads come in different sizes, and those 75–250 μm in size are frequently used for the treatment of liver cancer. This size range is far smaller than the size of Gelpart embolic agents (1,000 μm). Accordingly, the goal of arterial embolization in liver cancer today is to fill the blood vessels inside the tumor and the nearby tissues with embolic materials, instead of performing proximal embolization to block blood supply to the tumor as in the conventional embolization method. As shown in the PRECISION V randomized clinical study in 2010 [77, 78], treatment outcomes are similar between DEB-TACE and cTACE, but DEB-TACE is associated with fewer side effects. However, if a similar comparative trial were conducted in Japan, where cTACE is performed, using superselective techniques, cTACE may turn out to be superior in terms of validity. Regardless of such a study's results, there are a number of issues with DEB-TACE that need to be addressed. Well-organized clinical trials are necessary to answer questions regarding the selection DEB-TACE over cTACE and the effectiveness of DEB-TACE in patients who do not respond to cTACE.

Another technique that has been attracting attention is the balloon-occluded TACE (B-TACE) [79]. The principle of B-TACE is that when the blood pressure of the hepatic artery, which supplies normal liver parenchyma, drops distal to the balloon occlusion site, the flow of lipiodol declines quickly due to the narrow diameter of the arterial branches. In contrast, the amount of lipiodol flowing into the tumor increases because of the wide diameter of the vessels supplying the tumor. Subsequently, all the blood vessels supplying the tumor are blocked, and they become molded by continuously injecting embolic agents into them even after the flow in the tumor vessels is reduced to almost none and by moving the embolic agents into collateral blood vessels via the portal vein, which functions as a drainage vessel from the tumor. B-TACE is therefore a unique technique. Although it was reported to embolize target tumors effectively [79], further study is needed to verify this. Also, attracting attention is FlightPlan, which uses cone-beam CT to identify tumor vessels, but at present FlightPlan is limited to certain facilities because it requires special equipment and software.

Outside Japan, transarterial radioembolization is being frequently performed [80, 81]. Its introduction to Japan is eagerly awaited.

Hepatic Arterial Infusion Chemotherapy

From a global perspective, systemic chemotherapies using cytotoxic anticancer agents seldom offer survival benefits. In Japan, hepatic arterial infusion chemotherapy (HAIC) accounts for 90% of the chemotherapies for liver cancer. Two regimens are currently used in HAIC: low-dose 5-fluorouracil and cisplatin (FP) and IFN combined with 5-fluorouracil (IFN-5FU) [82]. It is difficult to compare the efficacy of each regimen because of the differences in the characteristics of patients and detailed protocols. According to Nouso et al. [83], a nationwide follow-up survey conducted by the Liver Cancer Study Group of Japan (LCSGJ) revealed excellent treatment outcomes for HAIC with low-dose FP, with a 40.5% response rate and median survival time of 16 months. On the other hand, the complete and partial response rates ranged widely from 25 to 63% in HAIC with IFN-5FU.

In the United States and Europe, HAIC is practically not performed because no prospective comparative clinical trials of HAIC have ever been done to produce any evidence of its efficacy. In Japan, however, the main problem associated with HAIC is whether advanced liver cancer should be treated first with sorafenib or with HAIC. Although prospective clinical trials are needed to demonstrate clear-cut evidence for HAIC in Western countries, it is not ethically possible for Japanese physicians to conduct a clinical trial comparing HAIC with no therapy because of the obvious superiority of HAIC. Furthermore, it would likely be impossible to observe any differences in a head-to-head comparison of HAIC and sorafenib therapy given that such a clinical trial would need to be performed as a crossover study with overall survival as the end point because HAIC and sorafenib therapy are both standard treatment methods for HCC in Japan. For this reason, a research group supported by Japan's Ministry of Health, Labour and Welfare is currently conducting the SILIUS clinical trial to compare the efficacy of the standard treatment method of sorafenib with that of sorafenib combined with HAIC (low-dose FP; NCT No. 00933816). This trial may be able to demonstrate, albeit indirectly, the survival benefits of HAIC. In addition to HAIC, radiation therapy is a treatment choice for patients with portal venous tumor thrombosis [84, 85].

Molecular Targeted Therapy

At present, sorafenib is the only drug with proven survival benefits [86], based on the results of 2 large-scale RCTs: the sorafenib HCC assessment randomized protocol (SHARP) study [87] and a trial conducted in the Asia-Pacific region [88]. Although many clinical trials

Dig Dis 2015;33:780–790
DOI: 10.1159/000439103

have been conducted to investigate various first- and second-line treatments using molecular targeted drugs with or without a combination of TACE or in the adjuvant setting, they all failed [89]. Therefore, the results of currently ongoing trials – first-line treatment with lenvatinib, second-line treatment with regorafenib, tivantinib treatment in patients with a high expression of cMet, ramucirumab treatment in patients with a higher AFP level (≥400 ng/ml) and anti–PD-1 antibody – are eagerly awaited. Regardless of the results of these trials, there is an urgent need for us to have to 1 or 2 more molecular targeted agents effective for HCC, beyond just sorafenib, to improve the survival of HCC patients. Biomarker for predicting the response of targeted therapy is another important issue [90].

The most promising treatment strategy for HCC is the combined use of a targeted agent with a locoregional therapy [91, 92]. The results of the STORM trial that is investigating sorafenib as an adjuvant therapy after hepatectomy or RFA (which has produced negative results), the TACTICS trial (NCT No. 01217034) that is investigating the combination of sorafenib with TACE and the SILIUS trial (NCT No. 01214343) that is investigating the combination of sorafenib with HAIC are keenly awaited. Prevention of HCC [93] is another important issue.

Response Evaluation Criteria for Liver Cancer

The Response Evaluation Criteria in Solid Tumors (RECIST), modified RECIST (mRECIST) [94, 95] and the LCSGJ's Response Evaluation Criteria in Cancer of the Liver (RECICL) [10, 96] are available for treatment response evaluation in liver cancer. However, RECIST is not suitable for response evaluation of locoregional therapies such as ablation or TACE because the criteria were originally developed to evaluate tumor response to chemotherapy and because it is extremely rare for these locoregional therapies to reduce the size of HCC tumors [97]. Furthermore, even when a necrogenic effect is induced by chemotherapy, the effect cannot be evaluated using RECIST. Despite mRECIST having been developed to overcome the shortcomings of RECIST, mRECIST also utilizes 1-dimensional measurement and thus differs greatly from LCSGJ's RECICL. However, RECICL also has its shortcomings because it was originally developed based on criteria established for the evaluation of direct treatment response to locoregional therapy, such as TACE or ablation, and not to chemotherapy. Therefore, the problem with RECICL, which was published in 2009, is that it does not take into account metastasis to other organs. Revision of the response evaluation criteria in the General Rules for the Clinical and Pathological Study of Primary Liver Cancer developed by LCSGJ has been published [10, 98].

Treatment Algorithm

Treatment algorithms for HCC have been developed by the AASLD [5] and the EASL-European Organisation for Research and Treatment of Cancer (EORTC) [6]. Both algorithms fundamentally adhere to the Barcelona Clinic Liver Cancer (BCLC) treatment algorithm. Basically, the treatment algorithm issued by the APASL [23] is not very different from other treatment algorithms. The conciseness of the Evidence-based Treatment Algorithm from the Japan Society of Hepatology (JSH) [24] is appreciated, but it is somewhat unclear because of the placement in the footnotes of some descriptions, such as vascular invasion and distant metastasis. In JSH's Consensus-based Treatment Algorithm [26], treatment options in line with evidence-based guidelines are provided in parallel with treatment choices based on expert consensus and are presented under separate topics such as extrahepatic spread, hepatic functional reserve, vascular invasion and the size and number of tumors. This consensus-based treatment algorithm is currently being used by experts in clinical practice, who also combine the evidence-based treatment algorithm with treatment methods without such evidence. Therefore, prospective clinical trials are needed to fill the gap between evidence-based and consensus-based treatment algorithms. While locoregional therapy is recommended in JSH's consensus-based algorithm as an experimental treatment for Child-Pugh (CP) C liver cancer based on the previous publication [99, 100], best supportive care is recommended in the evidence-based treatment algorithm. For this reason, the Japan Liver Oncology Group is currently planning a clinical trial of patients with CP-C liver cancer (with a CP score of 10–11) and cancer stage meeting the Milan criteria in order to compare best supportive care and locoregional therapy (RFA or TACE).

Definition of TACE Failure/Refractoriness

JSH was the first to define HCC failure/refractoriness to TACE in 2010, in the Management of Hepatocellular Carcinoma in Japan: Consensus-Based Clinical Practice Manual [101] as well as in an article published in Digestive Diseases [102]. The definition was subsequently revised by LCSGJ in 2014 [25] as well as JSH clinical practice manual [103]. The introduction of sorafenib triggered global awareness of the need to define TACE failure/refractoriness. Conventionally, when no other options are available, TACE is performed repeatedly even when it is no longer effective. However, the benefit that patients receive from TACE is defined as a balance between the anticancer effect of TACE and the preservation of hepatic functional reserve. When TACE no longer offers an antitumor effect, its repeated use only needlessly reduces the functional reserve and, theoretically, it is time to switch to another treatment. Globally, the next treatment option would be sorafenib, but in Japan, HAIC may be another option. The revised definition of TACE failure/refractoriness that LCSGJ issued in 2014 [25], although requiring verification in future studies, is believed to be superior to the EASL's criteria, which recommend switching to sorafenib when HCC has not responded to TACE twice, or the criteria used in Korea, which define HCC as refractory when a second TACE is required within 6 months. Actually, a study investigating the validity of TACE treatment in Japan has been published and has found LCSGJ's criteria to be suitable [104–107].

Prognostic Staging

Physicians treating liver cancer should be aware of the different staging systems used for liver cancer: those for deciding treatment strategy and those for prognostic prediction. Although BCLC stages [108] are sometimes compared with scores from the Cancer of the Liver Italian Program (CLIP) or the Japan Integrated Staging (JIS) system [109], the CLIP and the JIS scoring systems are staging systems for predicting prognosis, not for determining treatment strategies. In addition, BCLC staging involves just ordinary, common-sense treatment strategies, so to speak. In Japan, curative treatment is always selected for patients with the best TNM and liver function status, TACE is selected for patients with a moderate status and HAIC or sorafenib is selected for patients with advanced disease. It goes without saying that the survival analysis of these patients using the Kaplan–Meier estimation produces good stratification. On the other hand, the use of staging systems for prognostic prediction allows for the prognosis of patients to be determined using scores for prognostic factors in daily clinical practice and for groups of patients with the same prognostic scores to be compared between different institutions. Notably, the JIS scoring system is reported to be superior to the CLIP scoring system [109]. The modified JIS system, which replaces the CP classification with a classification of liver damage severity [110], and the biomarker combined JIS score (bm-JIS Score), which includes the tumor markers of AFP, PIVKA-II and AFP-L3 [111], have also been reported. It is understandable, then, that bm-JIS is theoretically superior to the conventional JIS score. The BALAD Scoring system has also been developed and uses albumin, bilirubin and the 3 tumor markers of AFP, PIVKA-II and AFP-L3, but not tumor staging or the CP classification [112]. This is an excellent staging system in that only blood sampling is required to predict prognosis in liver cancer. In the future, it will be necessary to determine which staging systems are most effective to apply in individual cases. Recently, the Hong Kong staging system has been introduced [113].

Subclassification of HCC

Molecular classification is a well-recognized system of HCC subclassification that classifies HCC based on the presence/absence of stem cell features [114–116]. This subclassification is also useful in determining future treatment targets and strategies. In addition, the finding that prognosis is good even when OATP8 is expressed in moderately differentiated liver cancer (i.e. shows hyperintensity in the hepatocyte phase of EOB-MRI) indicates a subclass of HCC. Also, because patients with CK19-positive HCC having stem cell features have shown poor prognosis [117], these tumors may be classified into a different subclass of HCC. Actually, even tumor markers may be important indicators of subtypes of HCC. Therefore, future challenges are the establishment of proper HCC subclassification methods and the respective treatment strategies for each subtype of HCC.

Conclusion

The current challenges and future prospects of clinical research on HCC have been reviewed. It is probably correct to say that, at the present, Japan greatly outperforms other countries in clinical practices for the disease, and emphasis should be placed on continuing to perform high-quality clinical studies such as multicenter, prospective comparative clinical trials in a straightforward manner.

Disclosure Statement

Authors declare no conflict of interest.

References

1 Kokudo N: Recent progress in the treatment and diagnosis of hepatocellular carcinoma. Liver Cancer 2013;2:4.

2 Kudo M: Alpha-fetoprotein-L3: useful or useless for hepatocellular carcinoma? Liver Cancer 2013;2:151–152.

3 Song P, Gao J, Inagaki Y, Kokudo N, Hasegawa K, Sugawara Y, Tang W: Biomarkers: evaluation of screening for and early diagnosis of hepatocellular carcinoma in Japan and China. Liver Cancer 2013;2:31–39.

4 Toyoda H, Kumada T, Tada T, Sone Y, Kaneoka Y, Maeda A: Tumor markers for hepatocellular carcinoma: simple and significant predictors of outcome in patients with HCC. Liver Cancer 2015;4:126–136.

5 Bruix J, Sherman M; American Association for the Study of Liver Diseases: Management of hepatocellular carcinoma: an update. Hepatology 2011;53:1020–1022.

6 European Association for the Study of the Liver; European Organisation for Research and Treatment of Cancer: EASL-EORTC clinical practice guidelines: management of hepatocellular carcinoma. J Hepatol 2012;56: 908–943.

7 Clinical practice guidelines for hepatocellular carcinoma differ between Japan, United States, and Europe. Liver Cancer 2015;4:85–95.

8 Asahina Y, Tsuchiya K, Tamaki N, Hirayama I, Tanaka T, Sato M, Yasui Y, Hosokawa T, Ueda K, Kuzuya T, Nakanishi H, Itakura J, Takahashi Y, Kurosaki M, Enomoto N, Izumi N: Effect of aging on risk for hepatocellular carcinoma in chronic hepatitis C virus infection. Hepatology 2010;52:518–527.

9 Osaki Y, Ueda Y, Marusawa H, Nakajima J, Kimura T, Kita R, Nishikawa H, Saito S, Henmi S, Sakamoto A, Eso Y, Chiba T: Decrease in alpha-fetoprotein levels predicts reduced incidence of hepatocellular carcinoma in patients with hepatitis C virus infection receiving interferon therapy: a single center study. J Gastroenterol 2012;47:444–451.

10 Kudo M, Ueshima K, Kubo S, Sakamoto M, Tanaka M, Ikai I, Furuse J, Murakami T, Kadoya M, Kokudo N: Response evaluation criteria in cancer of the liver (RECICL) (2015 revised version). Hepatol Res 2015, Epub ahead of print.

11 Koike Y, Shiratori Y, Sato S, Obi S, Teratani T, Imamura M, Yoshida H, Shiina S, Omata M: Des-gamma-carboxy prothrombin as a useful predisposing factor for the development of portal venous invasion in patients with hepatocellular carcinoma: a prospective analysis of 227 patients. Cancer 2001;91:561–569.

12 Mise Y, Sakamoto Y, Ishizawa T, Kaneko J, Aoki T, Hasegawa K, Sugawara Y, Kokudo N: A worldwide survey of the current daily practice in liver surgery. Liver Cancer 2013;2:55–66.

13 Shindoh J, Kaseb A, Vauthey JN: Surgical strategy for liver cancers in the era of effective chemotherapy. Liver Cancer 2013;2:47–54.

14 Lin SM: Local ablation for hepatocellular carcinoma in Taiwan. Liver Cancer 2013;2:73–83.

15 Teng W, Liu KW, Lin CC, Jeng WJ, Chen WT, Sheen IS, Lin CY, Lin SM: Insufficient ablative margin determined by early computed tomography may predict the recurrence of hepatocellular carcinoma after radiofrequency ablation. Liver Cancer 2015;4:26–38.

16 Yoshida H, Shiratori Y, Kudo M, Shiina S, Mizuta T, Kojiro M, Yamamoto K, Koike Y, Saito K, Koyanagi N, Kawabe T, Kawazoe S, Kobashi H, Kasugai H, Osaki Y, Araki Y, Izumi N, Oka H, Tsuji K, Toyota J, Seki T, Osawa T, Masaki N, Ichinose M, Seike M, Ishikawa A, Ueno Y, Tagawa K, Kuromatsu R, Sakisaka S, Ikeda H, Kuroda H, Kokuryu H, Yamashita T, Sakaida I, Katamoto T, Kikuchi K, Nomoto M, Omata M: Effect of vitamin K2 on the recurrence of hepatocellular carcinoma. Hepatology 2011;54:532–540.

17 Ueshima K, Kudo M, Takita M, Nagai T, Tatsumi C, Ueda T, Kitai S, Ishikawa E, Yada N, Inoue T, Hagiwara S, Minami Y, Chung H, Sakurai T: Des-γ-carboxyprothrombin may be a promising biomarker to determine the therapeutic efficacy of sorafenib for hepatocellular carcinoma. Dig Dis 2011;29:321–325.

18 Peck-Radosavljevic M: Drug therapy for advanced-stage liver cancer. Liver Cancer 2014; 3:125–131.

19 Siegel AB, El-Khoueiry AB, Finn RS, Guthrie KA, Goyal A, Venook AP, Blanke CD, Verna EC, Dove L, Emond J, Kato T, Samstein B, Busuttil R, Remotti H, Coffey A, Brown RS Jr: Phase I trial of sorafenib following liver transplantation in patients with high-risk hepatocellular carcinoma. Liver Cancer 2015;4:115–125.

20 Kumada T, Toyoda H, Tada T, Kiriyama S, Tanikawa M, Hisanaga Y, Kanamori A, Tanaka J, Kagebayashi C, Satomura S: High-sensitivity Lens culinaris agglutinin-reactive alpha-fetoprotein assay predicts early detection of hepatocellular carcinoma. J Gastroenterol 2014;49:555–563.

21 Tamura Y, Igarashi M, Kawai H, Suda T, Satomura S, Aoyagi Y: Clinical advantage of highly sensitive on-chip immunoassay for fucosylated fraction of alpha-fetoprotein in patients with hepatocellular carcinoma. Dig Dis Sci 2010;55:3576–3583.

22 Toyoda H, Kumada T, Tada T, Ito T, Maeda A, Kaneoka Y, Kagebayashi C, Satomura S: Changes in highly sensitive alpha-fetoprotein for the prediction of the outcome in patients with hepatocellular carcinoma after hepatectomy. Cancer Med 2014;3:643–651.

23 Omata M, Lesmana LA, Tateishi R, Chen PJ, Lin SM, Yoshida H, Kudo M, Lee JM, Choi BI, Poon RT, Shiina S, Cheng AL, Jia JD, Obi S, Han KH, Jafri W, Chow P, Lim SG, Chawla YK, Budihusodo U, Gani RA, Lesmana CR, Putranto TA, Liaw YF, Sarin SK: Asian Pacific association for the study of the liver consensus recommendations on hepatocellular carcinoma. Hepatol Int 2010;4:439–474.

24 Japan Society of Hepatology: Evidence-Based Clinical Practice Guidelines for Hepatocellular Carcinoma. Tokyo, Kanehara & Co., 2013.

25 Kudo M, Matsui O, Izumi N, Iijima H, Kadoya M, Imai Y, Okusaka T, Miyayama S, Tsuchiya K, Ueshima K, Hiraoka A, Ikeda M, Ogasawara S, Yamashita T, Minami T, Yamakado K; Liver Cancer Study Group of Japan: JSH consensus-based clinical practice guidelines for the management of hepatocellular carcinoma: 2014 update by the Liver Cancer Study Group of Japan. Liver Cancer 2014;3:458–468.

26 Kudo M, Hatanaka K, Maekawa K: Newly developed novel ultrasound technique, defect reperfusion ultrasound imaging, using sonazoid in the management of hepatocellular carcinoma. Oncology 2010;78(suppl 1):40–45.

27 Kudo M, Hatanaka K, Kumada T, Toyoda H, Tada T: Double-contrast ultrasound: a novel surveillance tool for hepatocellular carcinoma. Am J Gastroenterol 2011;106:368–370.

28 Kudo M, Hatanaka K, Chung H, Minami Y, Maekawa K: A proposal of novel treatment-assist technique for hepatocellular carcinoma in the Sonazoid-enhanced ultrasonography: value of defect re-perfusion imaging. Kanzo 2007;48:299–301.

29 Yada N, Kudo M, Morikawa H, Fujimoto K, Kato M, Kawada N: Assessment of liver fibrosis with real-time tissue elastography in chronic viral hepatitis. Oncology 2013;84 (suppl 1):13–20.

30 Kudo M: Prediction of hepatocellular carcinoma incidence risk by ultrasound elastography. Liver Cancer 2014;3:1–5.

31 Sakurai T, Kudo M: Molecular link between liver fibrosis and hepatocellular carcinoma. Liver Cancer 2013;2:365–366.

32 Ramakrishna G, Rastogi A, Trehanpati N, Sen B, Khosla R, Sarin SK: From cirrhosis to hepatocellular carcinoma: new molecular insights on inflammation and cellular senescence. Liver Cancer 2013;2:367–383.

33 Hsu C, Chen BB, Chen CH, Ho MC, Cheng JC, Kokudo N, Murakami T, Yeo W, Seong J, Jia JD, Han KH, Cheng AL: Consensus development from the 5th Asia-Pacific primary liver cancer expert meeting (APPLE 2014). Liver Cancer 2015;4:96–105.

34 Kudo M, Matsui O, Sakamoto M, Kitao A, Kim T, Ariizumi S, Ichikawa T, Kobayashi S, Imai Y, Izumi N, Fujinaga Y, Arii S: Role of gadolinium-ethoxybenzyl-diethylenetriamine pentaacetic acid-enhanced magnetic resonance imaging in the management of hepatocellular carcinoma: consensus at the symposium of the 48th annual meeting of the Liver Cancer Study Group of Japan. Oncology 2013;84(suppl 1):21–27.

35 Ichikawa T, Sano K, Morisaka H: Diagnosis of pathologically early HCC with EOB-MRI: experiences and current consensus. Liver Cancer 2014;3:97–107.

36 Kudo M: Early hepatocellular carcinoma: definition and diagnosis. Liver Cancer 2013;2: 69–72.
37 Kudo M: Surveillance, diagnosis, treatment, and outcome of liver cancer in Japan. Liver Cancer 2015;4:39–50.
38 Matsuda M, Tsuda T, Yoshioka S, Murata S, Tanaka H, Hirooka M, Hiasa Y, Mochizuki T: Incidence for progression of hypervascular HCC in hypovascular hepatic nodules showing hyperintensity on gadoxetic acid-enhanced hepatobiliary phase in patients with chronic liver diseases. Jpn J Radiol 2014;32:405–413.
39 Jang KM, Kim SH, Kim YK, Choi D: Imaging features of subcentimeter hypointense nodules on gadoxetic acid-enhanced hepatobiliary phase MR imaging that progress to hypervascular hepatocellular carcinoma in patients with chronic liver disease. Acta Radiol 2015; 56:526–535.
40 Komatsu N, Motosugi U, Maekawa S, Shindo K, Sakamoto M, Sato M, Tatsumi A, Miura M, Amemiya F, Nakayama Y, Inoue T, Fukasawa M, Uetake T, Ohtaka M, Sato T, Asahina Y, Kurosaki M, Izumi N, Ichikawa T, Araki T, Enomoto N: Hepatocellular carcinoma risk assessment using gadoxetic acid-enhanced hepatocyte phase magnetic resonance imaging. Hepatol Res 2014;44:1339–1346.
41 Iannicelli E, Di Pietropaolo M, Marignani M, Briani C, Federici GF, Delle Fave G, David V: Gadoxetic acid-enhanced MRI for hepatocellular carcinoma and hypointense nodule observed in the hepatobiliary phase. Radiol Med 2014;119:367–376.
42 Inoue T, Hyodo T, Murakami T, Takayama Y, Nishie A, Higaki A, Korenaga K, Sakamoto A, Osaki Y, Aikata H, Chayama K, Suda T, Takano T, Miyoshi K, Koda M, Numata K, Tanaka H, Iijima H, Ochi H, Hirooka M, Imai Y, Kudo M: Hypovascular hepatic nodules showing hypointense on the hepatobiliary-phase image of Gd-EOB-DTPA-enhanced MRI to develop a hypervascular hepatocellular carcinoma: a nationwide retrospective study on their natural course and risk factors. Dig Dis 2013;31:472–479.
43 Ichikawa S, Ichikawa T, Motosugi U, Sano K, Morisaka H, Enomoto N, Matsuda M, Fujii H, Araki T: Presence of a hypovascular hepatic nodule showing hypointensity on hepatocyte-phase image is a risk factor for hypervascular hepatocellular carcinoma. J Magn Reson Imaging 2014;39:293–297.
44 Toyoda H, Kumada T, Tada T, Niinomi T, Ito T, Sone Y, Kaneoka Y, Maeda A: Non-hypervascular hypointense nodules detected by Gd-EOB-DTPA-enhanced MRI are a risk factor for recurrence of HCC after hepatectomy. J Hepatol 2013;58:1174–1180.
45 Hyodo T, Murakami T, Imai Y, Okada M, Hori M, Kagawa Y, Kogita S, Kumano S, Kudo M, Mochizuki T: Hypovascular nodules in patients with chronic liver disease: risk factors for development of hypervascular hepatocellular carcinoma. Radiology 2013;266: 480–490.
46 Kim YK, Lee WJ, Park MJ, Kim SH, Rhim H, Choi D: Hypovascular hypointense nodules on hepatobiliary phase gadoxetic acid-enhanced MR images in patients with cirrhosis: potential of DW imaging in predicting progression to hypervascular HCC. Radiology 2012;265:104–114.
47 Kobayashi S, Matsui O, Gabata T, Koda W, Minami T, Ryu Y, Kozaka K, Kitao A: Intranodular signal intensity analysis of hypovascular high-risk borderline lesions of HCC that illustrate multi-step hepatocarcinogenesis within the nodule on Gd-EOB-DTPA-enhanced MRI. Eur J Radiol 2012;81:3839–3845.
48 Kobayashi S, Matsui O, Gabata T, Koda W, Minami T, Ryu Y, Kozaka K, Kitao A: Relationship between signal intensity on hepatobiliary phase of gadolinium ethoxybenzyl diethylenetriaminepentaacetic acid (Gd-EOB-DTPA)-enhanced MR imaging and prognosis of borderline lesions of hepatocellular carcinoma. Eur J Radiol 2012;81:3002–3009.
49 Kobayashi S, Matsui O, Gabata T, Koda W, Minami T, Ryu Y, Kawai K, Kozaka K: Gadolinium ethoxybenzyl diethylenetriamine pentaacetic acid-enhanced magnetic resonance imaging findings of borderline lesions at high risk for progression to hypervascular classic hepatocellular carcinoma. J Comput Assist Tomogr 2011;35:181–186.
50 Joishi D, Ueno A, Tanimoto A, Okuda S, Masugi Y, Emoto K, Okuma K, Sakamoto M, Imai Y, Kuribayashi S: Natural course of hypovascular nodules detected on gadoxetic acid-enhanced MR imaging: presence of fat is a risk factor for hypervascularization. Magn Reson Med Sci 2013;12:281–287.
51 Motosugi U: Hypovascular hypointense nodules on hepatocyte phase gadoxetic acid-enhanced MR images: too early or too progressed to determine hypervascularity. Radiology 2013;267:317–318.
52 Takechi M, Tsuda T, Yoshioka S, Murata S, Tanaka H, Hirooka M, Mochizuki T: Risk of hypervascularization in small hypovascular hepatic nodules showing hypointense in the hepatobiliary phase of gadoxetic acid-enhanced MRI in patients with chronic liver disease. Jpn J Radiol 2012;30:743–751.
53 Takayama Y, Nishie A, Nakayama T, Asayama Y, Ishigami K, Kakihara D, Ushijima Y, Fujita N, Hirakawa M, Honda H: Hypovascular hepatic nodule showing hypointensity in the hepatobiliary phase of gadoxetic acid-enhanced MRI in patients with chronic liver disease: prediction of malignant transformation. Eur J Radiol 2012;81:3072–3078.
54 Akai H, Matsuda I, Kiryu S, Tajima T, Takao H, Watanabe Y, Imamura H, Kokudo N, Akahane M, Ohtomo K: Fate of hypointense lesions on Gd-EOB-DTPA-enhanced magnetic resonance imaging. Eur J Radiol 2012;81: 2973–2977.
55 Motosugi U, Ichikawa T, Sano K, Sou H, Onohara K, Muhi A, Amemiya F, Enomoto N, Matsuda M, Fujii H, Araki T: Outcome of hypovascular hepatic nodules revealing no gadoxetic acid uptake in patients with chronic liver disease. J Magn Reson Imaging 2011;34: 88–94.
56 Kumada T, Toyoda H, Tada T, Sone Y, Fujimori M, Ogawa S, Ishikawa T: Evolution of hypointense hepatocellular nodules observed only in the hepatobiliary phase of gadoxetate disodium-enhanced MRI. AJR Am J Roentgenol 2011;197:58–63.
57 Narita M, Hatano E, Arizono S, Miyagawa-Hayashino A, Isoda H, Kitamura K, Taura K, Yasuchika K, Nitta T, Ikai I, Uemoto S: Expression of OATP1B3 determines uptake of Gd-EOB-DTPA in hepatocellular carcinoma. J Gastroenterol 2009;44:793–798.
58 Kitao A, Matsui O, Yoneda N, Kozaka K, Shinmura R, Koda W, Kobayashi S, Gabata T, Zen Y, Yamashita T, Kaneko S, Nakanuma Y: The uptake transporter OATP8 expression decreases during multistep hepatocarcinogenesis: correlation with gadoxetic acid enhanced MR imaging. Eur Radiol 2011;21: 2056–2066.
59 Kitao A, Matsui O, Yoneda N, Kozaka K, Kobayashi S, Koda W, Gabata T, Yamashita T, Kaneko S, Nakanuma Y, Kita R, Arii S: Hypervascular hepatocellular carcinoma: correlation between biologic features and signal intensity on gadoxetic acid-enhanced MR images. Radiology 2012;265:780–789.
60 Yoneda N, Matsui O, Kitao A, Kita R, Kozaka K, Koda W, Kobayashi S, Gabata T, Ikeda H, Nakanuma Y: Hypervascular hepatocellular carcinomas showing hyperintensity on hepatobiliary phase of gadoxetic acid-enhanced magnetic resonance imaging: a possible subtype with mature hepatocyte nature. Jpn J Radiol 2013;31:480–490.
61 Yoneda N, Matsui O, Kitao A, Kozaka K, Gabata T, Sasaki M, Nakanuma Y, Murata K, Tani T: Beta-catenin-activated hepatocellular adenoma showing hyperintensity on hepatobiliary-phase gadoxetic-enhanced magnetic resonance imaging and overexpression of OATP8. Jpn J Radiol 2012;30:777–782.
62 Yamashita T, Forgues M, Wang W, Kim JW, Ye Q, Jia H, Budhu A, Zanetti KA, Chen Y, Qin LX, Tang ZY, Wang XW: EpCAM and alpha-fetoprotein expression defines novel prognostic subtypes of hepatocellular carcinoma. Cancer Res 2008;68:1451–1461.
63 Yamashita T, Kitao A, Matsui O, Hayashi T, Nio K, Kondo M, Ohno N, Miyati T, Okada H, Yamashita T, Mizukoshi E, Honda M, Nakanuma Y, Takamura H, Ohta T, Nakamoto Y, Yamamoto M, Takayama T, Arii S, Wang X, Kaneko S: Gd-EOB-DTPA-enhanced magnetic resonance imaging and alpha-fetoprotein predict prognosis of early-stage hepatocellular carcinoma. Hepatology 2014;60:1674–1685.
64 Ueda K, Matsui O, Kawamori Y, Nakanuma Y, Kadoya M, Yoshikawa J, Gabata T, Nonomura A, Takashima T: Hypervascular hepatocellular carcinoma: evaluation of hemodynamics with dynamic CT during hepatic arteriography. Radiology 1998;206:161–166.

65 Murakami T, Tsurusaki M: Hypervascular benign and malignant liver tumors that require differentiation from hepatocellular carcinoma: key points of imaging diagnosis. Liver Cancer 2014;3:85–96.
66 Donadon M, Torzilli G: Intraoperative ultrasound in patients with hepatocellular carcinoma: from daily practice to future trends. Liver Cancer 2013;2:16–24.
67 Ishizawa T, Kokudo N: The beginning of a new era of digestive surgery guided by fluorescence imaging. Liver Cancer 2014;3:6–8.
68 Han HS, Yoon YS, Cho JY, Hwang DW: Laparoscopic liver resection for hepatocellular carcinoma: Korean experiences. Liver Cancer 2013;2:25–30.
69 Gumbs AA, Gayet B: Adopting Gayet's techniques of totally laparoscopic liver surgery in the United States. Liver Cancer 2013;2:5–15.
70 Kubo S, Takemura S, Sakata C, Urata Y, Uenishi T: Adjuvant therapy after curative resection for hepatocellular carcinoma associated with hepatitis virus. Liver Cancer 2013;2:40–46.
71 Chan SC, Sharr WW, Chan AC, Chok KS, Lo CM: Rescue living-donor liver transplantation for liver failure following hepatectomy for hepatocellular carcinoma. Liver Cancer 2013;2:332–337.
72 Chan SC: Liver transplantation for hepatocellular carcinoma. Liver Cancer 2013;2:338–344.
73 Akamatsu N, Sugawara Y, Kokudo N: Living donor liver transplantation for patients with hepatocellular carcinoma. Liver Cancer 2014;3:108–118.
74 Makino Y, Imai Y, Igura T, Hori M, Fukuda K, Sawai Y, Kogita S, Ohama H, Matsumoto Y, Nakahara M, Zushi S, Kurokawa M, Isotani K, Takamura M, Fujita N, Murakami T: Utility of computed tomography fusion imaging for the evaluation of the ablative margin of radiofrequency ablation for hepatocellular carcinoma and the correlation to local tumor progression. Hepatol Res 2013;43:950–958.
75 Minami Y, Yagyu Y, Murakami T, Kudo M: Tracking navigation imaging of transcatheter arterial chemoembolization for hepatocellular carcinoma using three-dimensional cone-beam CT angiography. Liver Cancer 2014;3:53–61.
76 Raoul JL, Gilabert M, Piana G: How to define transarterial chemoembolization failure or refractoriness: a European perspective. Liver Cancer 2014;3:119–124.
77 Vogl TJ, Lammer J, Lencioni R, Malagari K, Watkinson A, Pilleul F, Denys A, Lee C: Liver, gastrointestinal, and cardiac toxicity in intermediate hepatocellular carcinoma treated with PRECISION TACE with drug-eluting beads: results from the PRECISION V randomized trial. AJR Am J Roentgenol 2011;197:W562–W570.
78 Lammer J, Malagari K, Vogl T, Pilleul F, Denys A, Watkinson A, Pitton M, Sergent G, Pfammatter T, Terraz S, Benhamou Y, Avajon Y, Gruenberger T, Pomoni M, Langenberger H, Schuchmann M, Dumortier J, Mueller C, Chevallier P, Lencioni R; PRECISION V Investigators: Prospective randomized study of doxorubicin-eluting-bead embolization in the treatment of hepatocellular carcinoma: results of the PRECISION V study. Cardiovasc Intervent Radiol 2010;33:41–52.
79 Irie T, Kuramochi M, Takahashi N: Dense accumulation of lipiodol emulsion in hepatocellular carcinoma nodule during selective balloon-occluded transarterial chemoembolization: measurement of balloon-occluded arterial stump pressure. Cardiovasc Intervent Radiol 2013;36:706–713.
80 Khajornjiraphan N, Thu NA, Chow PK: Yttrium-90 microspheres: a review of its emerging clinical indications. Liver Cancer 2015;4:6–15.
81 Edeline J, Gilabert M, Garin E, Boucher E, Raoul JL: Yttrium-90 microsphere radioembolization for hepatocellular carcinoma. Liver Cancer 2015;4:16–25.
82 Kudo M: Treatment of advanced hepatocellular carcinoma with emphasis on hepatic arterial infusion chemotherapy and molecular targeted therapy. Liver Cancer 2012;1:62–70.
83 Nouso K, Miyahara K, Uchida D, Kuwaki K, Izumi N, Omata M, Ichida T, Kudo M, Ku Y, Kokudo N, Sakamoto M, Nakashima O, Takayama T, Matsui O, Matsuyama Y, Yamamoto K; Liver Cancer Study Group of Japan: Effect of hepatic arterial infusion chemotherapy of 5-fluorouracil and cisplatin for advanced hepatocellular carcinoma in the Nationwide survey of primary liver cancer in Japan. Br J Cancer 2013;109:1904–1907.
84 Lee DS, Seong J: Radiotherapeutic options for hepatocellular carcinoma with portal vein tumor thrombosis. Liver Cancer 2014;3:18–30.
85 Choi C, Choi GH, Kim TH, Tanaka M, Meng MB, Seong J: Multimodality management for Barcelona clinic liver cancer stage C hepatocellular carcinoma. Liver Cancer 2014;3:405–416.
86 Kudo M: Biomarkers and personalized sorafenib therapy. Liver Cancer 2014;3:399–404.
87 Llovet JM, Ricci S, Mazzaferro V, Hilgard P, Gane E, Blanc JF, de Oliveira AC, Santoro A, Raoul JL, Forner A, Schwartz M, Porta C, Zeuzem S, Bolondi L, Greten TF, Galle PR, Seitz JF, Borbath I, Häussinger D, Giannaris T, Shan M, Moscovici M, Voliotis D, Bruix J; SHARP Investigators Study Group: Sorafenib in advanced hepatocellular carcinoma. N Engl J Med 2008;359:378–390.
88 Cheng AL, Kang YK, Chen Z, Tsao CJ, Qin S, Kim JS, Luo R, Feng J, Ye S, Yang TS, Xu J, Sun Y, Liang H, Liu J, Wang J, Tak WY, Pan H, Burock K, Zou J, Voliotis D, Guan Z: Efficacy and safety of sorafenib in patients in the Asia-Pacific region with advanced hepatocellular carcinoma: a phase III randomised, double-blind, placebo-controlled trial. Lancet Oncol 2009;10:25–34.
89 Recent advances in bioinformatics reveal the molecular heterogeneity of hepatocellular carcinoma. Liver Cancer 2014;3:68–70.
90 Shao YY, Hsu CH, Cheng AL: Predictive biomarkers of antiangiogenic therapy for advanced hepatocellular carcinoma: where are we? Liver Cancer 2013;2:93–107.
91 Kim HY, Park JW: Clinical trials of combined molecular targeted therapy and locoregional therapy in hepatocellular carcinoma: past, present, and future. Liver Cancer 2014;3:9–17.
92 Shen YC, Lin ZZ, Hsu CH, Hsu C, Shao YY, Cheng AL: Clinical trials in hepatocellular carcinoma: an update. Liver Cancer 2013;2:345–364.
93 Kawanaka M, Nishino K, Nakamura J, Oka T, Urata N, Goto D, Suehiro M, Kawamoto H, Kudo M, Yamada G: Quantitative levels of hepatitis B virus DNA and surface antigen and the risk of hepatocellular carcinoma in patients with hepatitis B receiving long-term nucleos(t)ide analogue therapy. Liver Cancer 2014;3:41–52.
94 Lencioni R, Llovet JM: Modified RECIST (mRECIST) assessment for hepatocellular carcinoma. Semin Liver Dis 2010;30:52–60.
95 Raoul JL, Park JW, Kang YK, Finn RS, Kim JS, Yeo W, Polite BN, Chao Y, Walters I, Baudelet C, Lencioni R: Using modified RECIST and alpha-fetoprotein levels to assess treatment benefit in hepatocellular carcinoma. Liver Cancer 2014;3:439–450.
96 Kudo M, Kubo S, Takayasu K, Sakamoto M, Tanaka M, Ikai I, Furuse J, Nakamura K, Makuuchi M; Liver Cancer Study Group of Japan (Committee for Response Evaluation Criteria in Cancer of the Liver, Liver Cancer Study Group of Japan): Response evaluation criteria in cancer of the liver (RECICL) proposed by the Liver Cancer Study Group of Japan (2009 revised version). Hepatol Res 2010;40:686–692.
97 Minami Y, Kudo M: Imaging modalities for assessment of treatment response to nonsurgical hepatocellular carcinoma therapy: contrast-enhanced US, CT, and MRI. Liver Cancer 2015;4:106–114.
98 The Liver Cancer Study Group of Japan: The General Rules for the Clinical and Pathological Study of Primary Liver Cancer, ed 6. Tokyo, Kanehara, 2015.
99 Nouso K, Ito Y, Kuwaki K, Kobayashi Y, Nakamura S, Ohashi Y, Yamamoto K: Prognostic factors and treatment effects for hepatocellular carcinoma in Child C cirrhosis. Br J Cancer 2008;98:1161–1165.
100 Kudo M, Osaki Y, Matsunaga T, Kasugai H, Oka H, Seki T: Hepatocellular carcinoma in Child-Pugh C cirrhosis: prognostic factors and survival benefit of nontransplant treatments. Dig Dis 2013;31:490–498.
101 Japan Society of Hepatology: Consensus-Based Clinical Practice Manual of Hepatocellular Carcinoma, ed 2. Tokyo, Igakushoin, 2010.

102 Kudo M, Izumi N, Kokudo N, Matsui O, Sakamoto M, Nakashima O, Kojiro M, Makuuchi M; HCC Expert Panel of Japan Society of Hepatology: Management of hepatocellular carcinoma in Japan: consensus-based clinical practice guidelines proposed by the Japan Society of Hepatology (JSH) 2010 updated version. Dig Dis 2011;29:339–364.

103 Japan Society of Hepatology: Management of Hepatocellular Carcinoma in Japan: Consensus-Based Clinical Practice Manual, ed 3. Tokyo, Igaku-Shoin, 2015.

104 Arizumi T, Ueshima K, Chishina H, Kono M, Takita M, Kitai S, Inoue T, Yada N, Hagiwara S, Minami Y, Sakurai T, Nishida N, Kudo M: Validation of the criteria of transcatheter arterial chemoembolization failure or refractoriness in patients with advanced hepatocellular carcinoma proposed by the LCSGJ. Oncology 2014;87(suppl 1):32–36.

105 Ogasawara S, Chiba T, Ooka Y, Kanogawa N, Motoyama T, Suzuki E, Tawada A, Kanai F, Yoshikawa M, Yokosuka O: Efficacy of sorafenib in intermediate-stage hepatocellular carcinoma patients refractory to transarterial chemoembolization. Oncology 2014;87:330–341.

106 Kudo M, Matsui O, Izumi N, Kadoya M, Okusaka T, Miyayama S, Yamakado K, Tsuchiya K, Ueshima K, Hiraoka A, Ikeda M, Ogasawara S, Yamashita T, Minami T; Liver Cancer Study Group of Japan: Transarterial chemoembolization failure/refractoriness: JSH-LCSGJ criteria 2014 update. Oncology 2014;87(suppl 1):22–31.

107 Arizumi T, Ueshima K, Minami T, Kono M, Chishina H, Takita M, Kitai S, Inoue T, Yada N, Hagiwara S, Minami Y, Sakurai T, Nishida N, Kudo M: Effectiveness of sorafenib in patients with transcatheter arterial chemoembolozation (TACE) refractory and intermediate-stage hepatocellular carcinoma. Liver Cancer 2015, in press.

108 Llovet JM, Brú C, Bruix J: Prognosis of hepatocellular carcinoma: the BCLC staging classification. Semin Liver Dis 1999;19:329–338.

109 Kudo M, Chung H, Haji S, Osaki Y, Oka H, Seki T, Kasugai H, Sasaki Y, Matsunaga T: Validation of a new prognostic staging system for hepatocellular carcinoma: the JIS score compared with the CLIP score. Hepatology 2004;40:1396–1405.

110 Ikai I, Takayasu K, Omata M, Okita K, Nakanuma Y, Matsuyama Y, Makuuchi M, Kojiro M, Ichida T, Arii S, Yamaoka Y; Liver Cancer Study Group of Japan: A modified Japan integrated stage score for prognostic assessment in patients with hepatocellular carcinoma. J Gastroenterol 2006;41:884–892.

111 Kitai S, Kudo M, Minami Y, Ueshima K, Chung H, Hagiwara S, Inoue T, Ishikawa E, Takahashi S, Asakuma Y, Haji S, Osaki Y, Oka H, Seki T, Kasugai H, Sasaki Y, Matsunaga T: A new prognostic staging system for hepatocellular carcinoma: value of the biomarker combined Japan integrated staging score. Intervirology 2008;51:86–94.

112 Toyoda H, Kumada T, Osaki Y, Oka H, Urano F, Kudo M, Matsunaga T: Staging hepatocellular carcinoma by a novel scoring system (BALAD score) based on serum markers. Clin Gastroenterol Hepatol 2006;4:1528–1536.

113 Poon RT, Cheung TT, Kwok PC, Lee AS, Li TW, Loke KL, Chan SL, Cheung MT, Lai TW, Cheung CC, Cheung FY, Loo CK, But YK, Hsu SJ, Yu SC, Yau T: Hong Kong consensus recommendations on the management of hepatocellular carcinoma. Liver Cancer 2015;4:51–69.

114 Hoshida Y, Toffanin S, Lachenmayer A, Villanueva A, Minguez B, Llovet JM: Molecular classification and novel targets in hepatocellular carcinoma: recent advancements. Semin Liver Dis 2010;30:35–51.

115 Lo RC, Ng IO: Hepatic progenitor cells: their role and functional significance in the new classification of primary liver cancers. Liver Cancer 2013;2:84–92.

116 Oishi N, Yamashita T, Kaneko S: Molecular biology of liver cancer stem cells. Liver Cancer 2014;3:71–84.

117 Tsuchiya K, Komuta M, Yasui Y, Tamaki N, Hosokawa T, Ueda K, Kuzuya T, Itakura J, Nakanishi H, Takahashi Y, Kurosaki M, Asahina Y, Enomoto N, Sakamoto M, Izumi N: Expression of keratin 19 is related to high recurrence of hepatocellular carcinoma after radiofrequency ablation. Oncology 2011;80:278–288.

Author Index Vol. 33, No. 6, 2015

Digestive Diseases

E-Mail karger@karger.com
www.karger.com/ddi

Subject Index Vol. 33, No. 6, 2015

Digestive Diseases

KARGER 125

E-Mail karger@karger.com
www.karger.com/ddi

Vol. 33, 2015

Digestive Diseases

Clinical Reviews

Formerly 'Survey of Digestive Diseases'
Founded in 1983 by T.S.N. Chen and R.K. Zetterman
Former Editor: S.R. Achem (1993–2000)

KARGER 125 YEARS

Basel • Freiburg • Paris • London • New York • Chennai • New Delhi • Bangkok • Beijing • Shanghai • Tokyo • Kuala Lumpur • Singapore • Sydney

Contents Vol. 33, 2015

Digestive Diseases

No. 1

Challenges in Inflammatory, Preneoplastic and Neoplastic Diseases of the Digestive System
Editor: Malfertheiner, P. (Magdeburg)

No. 2

Falk Symposium 193
Amsterdam, September 2014
Celiac Disease and Other Small Bowel Disorders
Editors: Mulder, C.J.J. (Amsterdam); Schuppan; D. (Mainz)

KARGER

E-Mail karger@karger.com
www.karger.com

Access to full text and tables of contents, including tentative ones for forthcoming issues:
www.karger.com/ddi_issues

No. 3

Falk Symposium 194
Freiburg, October 2014
Bile Acids as Signal Integrators and Metabolic Modulators
23rd International Bile Acid Meeting
Editors: Häussinger, D. (Düsseldorf); Beuers, U. (Amsterdam); Keitel, V. (Düsseldorf); Trauner, M. (Vienna)

S. Karger
Medical and Scientific Publishers
Basel • Freiburg • Paris • London •
New York • Chennai • New Delhi •
Bangkok • Beijing • Shanghai • Tokyo •
Kuala Lumpur • Singapore • Sydney

• Journal Publication

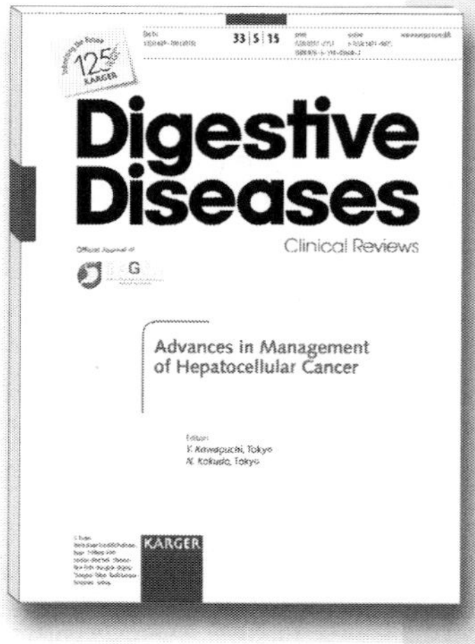

Advances in Management of Hepatocellular Cancer

Editors
Yoshikuni Kawaguchi
Norihiro Kokudo

Advances in Management of Hepatocellular Cancer
Editors: Kawaguchi, Y.; Kokudo, N. (Tokyo)
72 p., 21 fig., 5 in color, 9 tab., 2015
CHF 43.00 / EUR 40.00 / USD 51.00 (soft cover)
CHF 52.00 / EUR 48.00 / USD 61.00 (online)
Online version for institutional purchase
Prices subject to change, VAT not included
EUR price for eurozone countries, USD price for USA and Latin America only
ISBN 978-3-318-05607-5 (soft cover)
e-ISBN 978-3-318-05608-2

Special Topic Issue
Digestive Diseases
Vol. 33, No. 5 (2015)
Included in subscription

Listed in MEDLINE/PubMed

Contents

Dear Librarian

I have reviewed this publication and would like to recommend it for our library.

Recommended by:

Department:

Date:

Signature:

Orders may be placed with any bookshop, subscription agency, directly with the publisher or through a Karger distributor.

The easiest way to order: **www.karger.com/ddi**

Karger – Medical and Scientific Publishers
CH–4009 Basel, Switzerland
orders@karger.com, f: +41 61 306 12 34
www.karger.com

KI15426

KARGER